HEALTH OF THE STATE

Paul Adams

FOREWORD BY S.M. Miller

PRAEGER SPECIAL STUDIES IN SOCIAL WELFARE

GENERAL EDITORS:
Neil Gilbert and Harry Specht

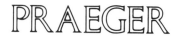

PRAEGER SPECIAL STUDIES • PRAEGER SCIENTIFIC

Library of Congress Cataloging in Publication Data

Adams, Paul
    Health of the state.

    (Praeger studies in social welfare)
    Bibliography: p.
    Includes index.
    1. War—Medical aspects.   2. War and society.
3. Medical policy—United States.   4. Medical
policy—Great Britain.   5. United States—Social
policy.   6. Great Britain—Social policy.
I. Title.   II. Series.
RA646.A3   362.1'042   81-22647
ISBN 0-03-058628-3   AACR2

TO KRISTI

Published in 1982 by Praeger Publishers
CBS Educational and Professional Publishing
a Division of CBS Inc.
521 Fifth Avenue, New York, New York 10175, U.S.A.

© 1982 by Praeger Publishers

23456789   145   987654321

Printed in the United States of America

CONTENTS

FOREWORD
BY
S.M. Miller

The American skeptic Randolph Bourne declared that "war is the health of the state," meaning that war expands what states are allowed to do. In this important, readable book Paul Adams turns that statement on its side and investigates the ways in which health challenges the state in wartime. In three probing case studies of nutrition, tuberculosis control, and venereal disease control during World War II, Adams has creatively detailed the differences between the United States and the United Kingdom in responding to health challenges during wartime.

War, Adams shows, led to the vast expansion of social programs in both countries. Crisis, he argues more generally, promotes social programs. The expansion of social programs, which led to a welfare state in Britain (but not in America), is not the result of a Fabian or Democratic visible hand inexorably, pragmatically, and gently unfolding social rights and programs. Rather, economic and political need, the possibility of disturbing turmoil, or the need for loyalty, consensus, and work motivation are the motors of social programs.

The book appears at an interesting time in both countries. In Britain, Thatcherism is sharply curtailing welfare state programs. In the United States, Cold War II is the health of the military state but not of the welfare state. Vast military outlays are crowding out social programs. In both countries many wonder whether turmoil will grow and disrupt the plans to spur capitalism by shifting burdens to the poor and vulnerable sectors of society.

Adams does not address that question; he deals with that important turning point of World War II, which ushered in Keynesian economic demand management and Beveridge social safety nets. But important lessons can be drawn from his analysis of a period of

vi

expansion of social programs for the present time of their contraction.

Social programs expand when they are connected to a still broader and more urgently regarded purpose. The appeal of solidarity, work motivation, and morale during wartime can lead to social programs. Another incentive is the need to maintain the labor force so that it can work or so that social peace can be maintained. Social programs, then, are usually not a simple reflection of need and generosity, but of other more politically or economically compelling pressures.

Social programs work more effectively, i.e., expand and receive little criticism, when they do not conflict with cultural values about work or morality. Indeed, public attitudes are an important part of social policy, in that they affect not only the basic legislation but also the daily administration of programs.

A frequent contention is that good programs are underutilized. But, as Adams shows, when the British working classes had more money, they spent it to improve their nutrition. Underutilization usually is a myth.

The most important social programs are employment and income maintenance. Adams illustrates that indirect effects of these two on nutrition and mental health are more important than more narrowly oriented programs.

In contrast to those who contend that redistribution is a drag on the economy and does little good for its beneficiaries, Adams shows how a reduced food supply was redistributed to children, pregnant women, and those employed in arduous work, so that the average level of health and nutrition improved. Redistribution without growth can produce important, positive results.

Information is an important political issue and shapes what happens to social and economic programs. Reliable information and its appropriate interpretation are very scarce goods. Many crucial issues of values are debated in the form of statistical disagreements. As Adams points out, governments can creatively utilize bad statistics. Cost-of-living data are reappraised and recategorized when they show results that are unpalatable for governments. Currently, in the United States the home ownership component of the consumer price index will be changed radically in order to reduce price level increases through statistical decree. In World War II, the same concern with statistics on prices rising faster than pleased the government led to rechristening the cost-of-living index as a more restricted consumer price index. Not only is naming the game, but interpreting the data is even more important. Pierre Bourdieu has written of the "social capital" of those born into more privileged status in society; for a class, as a whole, knowledge of statistics and their manipulation is important "political capital."

Social programs frequently seem to have a common history. At first, the social need or problem is minimized. Then, it is classified as an individual problem, as with venereal disease in the United States or with Rowntree's "secondary poverty" arising from the misuse of income. Third, the argument becomes that of underutilization; the afflicted would not do the appropriate thing if they were offered the chance of aid. The problem consequently cannot be alleviated. Fourth, pressure or crisis pushes aside these objections and a program may be adopted. Fifth, it grows through ad hoc adjustments, which cause difficulties of unevenness, inequity, poverty traps, and overdiscretion or overregulation. Sixth, programs are sharply criticized as too expensive or ineffective. Since they do not touch the mainstreams of economic functioning, they can only partially succeed in their objectives. Some measure of failure is thus built into their history and functioning.

This formulation not only regularizes complex events, but may smack too much of the cynicism of a Randolph Bourne. Unfortunately, in the United States this last stage is a current reality. The Adams book helps us understand how we have come to our present state.

Adams also helps us to deepen our methodological approaches for the study of social policy. He writes in the tradition of political economy, which seeks to show how the state's activities are shaped by pressures to aid capitalist economic functioning while maintaining political legitimacy. His careful analyses make it possible to deepen and elaborate that approach, particularly by recognizing countertendencies, in at least five ways.

First, Adams stresses the differences between a "weak state" like the United States and a "strong state" like the United Kingdom. The United States has a much more decentralized form of government than the United Kingdom, making it much more difficult for Washington to exercise the influence and discretion that Whitehall can. A visible marker is the much higher proportion of total taxes collected by the U.K. central government compared to that percentage which flows to the U.S. federal government. Again, the United States is a weak state in that the government can exercise less power over activities than it can in the United Kingdom. The form and scope of the state are important in understanding what it does (and does not do).

Second, it is not easy for the state to operate in terms of the long-term interests of the capitalist class as a whole, a central tenet of some political economy approaches. What long-term interests are, is not easy to predict and act upon. Sectoral interests can block out efforts to act in terms of broad, long-run concerns. The ascendancy of one or another sector's interests may be very common indeed. As Adams shows, agricultural interest dominated food policy in the United States that in ways may have been deleterious to the war effort.

Third, social sector expenditures may benefit nonmonopoly sectors much more than monopoly sectors. This inference counters

James O'Connor's argument in <u>The Fiscal Crisis of the State</u> that the monopoly sector is the main beneficiary of the state's economic activity. Agricultural groups, in the wartime period when agribusiness did not predominate, were undoubtedly the prime shapers and beneficiaries of U.S. food policies.

Fourth, political culture and history mold much of what the state does. To ignore them is to encapsulate a wide range of experience into a very limited framework of economic determinism. Adams contrasts the very different ways that the United States and the United Kingdom faced the venereal disease threat. Because of the strong cultural (and consequently political) stress on moral principles, the United States found it difficult to maintain a policy of prevention and primary care of V.D. The United Kingdom's culture permitted greater adaptability in dealing with the possibilities of V.D.

Fifth, motivation and intent are only the first stages of policy. The evolution of policy and its outcomes must be separately and concretely analyzed. One cannot infer from motivation what the effects were, nor from effects describe intentions. Indeed, more than intentions, students of social policy may have to study how policies become reshaped during their lifetimes, with changing effects. Adams examines the initial preoccupation of United Kingdom food policy makers with containing price inflation by preventing contrived shortages; over time, the control over supply made possible the redistribution of food and the resulting improvement of general health. The important result was far distant from the initial preoccupation with prices.

These points do not invalidate the political economy approach, but fill it out, providing neglected nuances. Adams, of course, did not start out to make the points that have been drawn above, and might well object to them. But the beauty of this rich, detailed analysis is that it permits these and other important points to be made. One measure of excellent case studies is what they can stimulate in the way of theorizing. Adams has certainly met that test. In focusing on three case studies, Adams has made a significant contribution to understanding the evolution of social policies and their impact.

ACKNOWLEDGMENTS

For critical scrutiny of the manuscript in its several versions, and for many valuable comments and suggestions, I am grateful to James Leiby. Gary Freeman, Samuel R. Friedman, William Kornhauser, Clarence Lo, David Matza, S.M. Miller and J.M. Winter also read all or part of the manuscript and commented helpfully upon it. A special debt is due my wife, Kristine Nelson, whose critical and editorial advice improved the work greatly. Parts of Chapter One appeared in the Journal of Sociology and Social Welfare 4 (1977): 419-32.

1

INTRODUCTION

In all advanced capitalist countries, social welfare is primarily a state responsibility, and a major part of the state's activity. The state has met more and more of the capital costs of maintaining a labor force at an adequate level of health, education, and economic security, including provision for the risks of unemployment, disability, and old age. It has also taken over much of the social control function of social welfare, socializing the expenses of maintaining order and harmony.(1)

Collective provision for individual dependency and insecurity is sometimes seen as evolving "from poor law to welfare state," from "charity to social justice," resulting in an array of programs through which the state maintains "minimum standards of income, nutrition, health, housing, and education for every citizen, assured to him as political right, not as charity."(2) A secular trend in this direction is evident, certainly, but so is a countertendency, less powerful in the long run but of great importance nonetheless, toward "reprivatization" – the development of private alternatives to social provision, a shift to reliance on market mechanisms, and a cutting back of social welfare programs.(3)

In neither Britain nor the United States has the welfare state evolved in a smooth and continuous progression. Rather, like capitalism itself, the inner logic of which has given rise to remarkably similar "welfare states" in all the advanced countries, it has developed unevenly through a series of crises.

The major international crises of the present century, the two world wars and the Great Depression, have elicited new levels of state intervention in economic and social life. External and internal threats to the existing regime and to power relationships between classes have overcome resistance to an expansion of the state's role, even in the face of a strong antistatist tradition. Once the crisis is past, the pressures toward reprivatization reassert themselves, but a return to precrisis "normalcy" is no longer possible. The state's intervention produces economic, political, and ideological effects that rule out such a restoration. The crisis is a turning point.(4)

This study explores the impact of World War II on the state's intervention in certain areas of health policy in Britain and the United States. I begin by developing a general theory of the relationship between social policy, social class, and the state. Social policy is seen as pressed out between the needs of capital for a regulated supply of efficient labor power and for social order, on the one hand, and the pressure exerted by the working class (and specially oppressed groups) for decent standards of health, housing, education, and economic security, on the other. The state's mediation of these needs and pressures is explored in Chapter Two in the context of a discussion of the relation between war and social policy. Though central to an understanding of modern social welfare, the theory of the capitalist state has largely been ignored by even the more theoretically inclined social policy analysts.

War differs, as a crisis, from a major depression. In using the term crisis, somewhat loosely, I mean to focus on a "deep analogy" between periods in which everyday expectations break down, the existing ceases to seem inevitable or even viable, the status quo is in jeopardy.(5) In particular, a comparison and contrast between the Depression and World War II, as crises, pervades the study. They are not, of course, comparable as crises of accumulation, as fiscal crises, or as military crises. But seeing them as crises in a more general sense, closer to the medical usage from which the metaphor developed (that is, as examples of a turning point for better or worse in an acute disease or fever), enables us to focus on both the common features of those events and the different kinds of challenge they presented for the state and the existing social order.(6)

My aim is to contribute to the understanding of the nature and evolution of the welfare state, and at the same time to examine three specific areas of social policy and state interventionism in Britain and the United States. Nutrition, tuberculosis control, and venereal disease control were selected because of their significance for the nation's health. With manpower at a premium in all combatant countries, World War II made health a problem for the state. In the Depression, the fitness of the military and the industrial work force was not a central concern of the state's social policy. In World War II it was.

Wartime social policy concerns extended far beyond the fighters and war workers who contributed directly to the national struggle. Maternal and child health, and child welfare, for instance, were also considered important. In Britain right-wing conservatives supported family allowances, which further socialized the costs of child rearing, as part of a sound military strategy. Nutrition overlaps these policy areas, however, and has a representative quality in reflecting the state's concern for mothers and children, as well as for soldiers and war workers.

Nutrition was important because of its significance for general health and morale. As governments became involved in regulating and organizing national food supplies, they were increasingly drawn into questions of nutritional policy even where they would have preferred to ignore them. Ensuring adequate nutrition was closely tied to questions, not only of food policy, but also of prices and income control, questions of central importance to preserving peace during wartime inflation.

Control of tuberculosis and venereal disease, the other areas that I examine in detail, also assumed renewed importance for the state in war, for they were major drains on young, adult manpower. Both, moreover, tended to increase in war, and neither, at the beginning of World War II, was easily curable. Tuberculosis was closely linked with the general conditions of life of a population, incidence and prevalence being functions of income, nutrition, housing, and so forth. Venereal disease carried a strong moral stigma, and policies for its control reflected religious and moral traditions regarding the social control of sexual behavior.

Each of these policy areas was problematic for the state at war, and elicited new levels of state intervention in both Britain and America. Each is examined in terms of, and in the context of, a larger analysis of war and the welfare state. Each may be seen as a test of the applicability of the general framework to a specific area of social policy.

However, they are not illustrations or examples of the larger analysis. They are elements of the total picture, not small-scale versions of it. They are not necessarily expressive of the totality in the sense that a random sample represents the population from which it is taken.(7) Each has its own, relatively autonomous, history, and interacts differently with the economy, politics, and ideology of the social formation. Each social policy area is seen as an element of a larger structural unity in which the economic instance is ultimately decisive. Nutrition, being linked so closely with the whole management of the economy at war, may be expected to correspond more closely to the larger pattern. But venereal disease control, impinging less strongly on major capitalist interests, allows more room for the influence of ideology and tradition to be decisive. While the specific and general levels of analysis illuminate each other, therefore, it is not by way of one providing a microcosm of the other.

This is a comparative study. It involves the comparison not only of different crises and different social policy areas, but also of two different countries. Britain and the United States share much in common, in language, culture, politics, and economic system. There has always been a high level of interaction between them in the sphere of social welfare, as in other areas. Though they are sufficiently alike to make comparison meaningful, they entered World War II as significantly different social formations. The war itself had a strikingly different impact on each country (as did the Depression), but they differed at the outset in economic position, ideology, politics, and social structure.

In the crisis of total war, not only manpower, but also morale was at a premium. The state, relatively autonomous, but not independent, in relation to the balance of class forces, had to maintain national solidarity as well as ensure the fitness of its military and industrial manpower. This task was an important consideration of social policy both during the war and in the development of plans for the postwar world.

Many other areas of social policy and the welfare state remain unexplored in this study. In particular, maternal and child health, and the organization and financing of the health care system, need further investigation in terms of the kind of analysis developed here. What I offer is a preliminary application of a fruitful approach to the understanding of the welfare state. Historiographically, it provides a case for increased attention to World War II, largely ignored by American historians of social welfare, as a critical period in the development of the welfare state. It calls for attention to the importance of major crises in general, and especially wars, for the development of social welfare, and also to the necessity for developing an adequate theory of the state. The specific analyses of nutrition, and of tuberculosis and venereal disease control, indicate both the value and the complexities of examining concrete historical experience in the light of high-level generalizations or models of the kind developed by social scientists, and regarded with suspicion by many historians.

Policy-relevant investigations and reports that deal with the health care system or other aspects of social welfare often have essentially a symbolic function, despite their practical orientation. They give the appearance of suprapolitical rationality and technical expertise, while leaving deeply embedded structural problems and interests undisturbed.(8) Social workers, social policy analysts, and others who wish to change the social welfare system need to understand the nature and evolution of the welfare state. The structure and dynamics of social welfare in a modern capitalist state create certain objective possibilities for change and close off others. An effective strategy for change depends upon a grasp of the structural interests that act as barriers to genuine reform. It is also important to understand the contradictions generated by the system in the course of its development, and the inherent possibilities for change that they present.(9) This work is not directly concerned with strategy, and makes no policy proposals. But it aspires to contribute to the building of a knowledge base upon which effective strategy can be developed.

A word about usage. The pattern of health problems and state responses was somewhat different in Scotland from the rest of Britain. I do not attempt to provide the separate account that the Scottish experience sometimes requires. In general, "Britain" here refers to England and Wales when health patterns are under discussion, but to the United Kingdom of Great Britain and Northern Ireland when the national political entity is meant. In order to avoid both the awkwardness of discussing the "United States state" and the confusion of different levels of government ("United States" often meaning federal as distinct from state and local), I have retained the adjective "American," even though the United States is the only American country discussed here.

I have attempted to avoid sexist usage. To avert confusion, however, certain job classifications have been retained in the form they had in the 1930s and 1940s. I also decided to keep "manpower," after rejecting both "labor power," as inappropriate for the military at war, and "human-power," as sounding too human, that is, unalienated.

NOTES

(1)   Paul Adams, "Social Control or Social Wage," pp. 46-48; James O'Connor, Fiscal Crisis of the State, pp. 111-74.

(2)   Walter I. Trattner, From Poor Law to Welfare State; John M. Romanyshyn, Social Welfare: Charity to Justice; Harold Wilensky and Charles N. Lebeaux, Industrial Society and Social Welfare, p. xii.

(3)   Richard M. Titmuss, Social Policy, pp. 38-43.

(4)   Cf. Gunnar Myrdal, Beyond the Welfare State, pp. 24-29.

(5)   Arthur L. Stinchcombe, Theoretical Methods in Social History, pp. 19-22.

(6)   See Jurgen Habermas, Legitimation Crisis, pp. 1-31.

(7)   See Louis Althusser and Etienne Balibar, Reading Capital, p. 94; Alex Callinicos, Althusser's Marxism, pp. 39-52.

(8)   Robert R. Alford, Health Care Politics, p. 101; Murray Edelman, Symbolic Uses of Politics; Ida R. Hoos, Systems Analysis in Public Policy, pp. 109-10.

(9)   Sander Kelman, "Adventure in the Undialectical," p. 128.

2

SOCIAL POLICY AND WAR

American writers on social policy usually treat war as a diversion or interruption of progress toward a welfare state. The Progressive era was cut off by World War I, the New Deal was liquidated as a hostile Congress and an indifferent president turned their attention to World War II, and the War on Poverty gave way to the Vietnam War. "War," Max Lerner said in 1940, "generally puts an end to any period of social reform."(1) British writers, however, see it differently. Most have agreed with Maurice Bruce that the "decisive event in the evolution of the Welfare State was the Second World War. . . .The years of active thought and planning were those from 1941 to 1948: these mark an epoch in British history."(2) The difference suggests both the distinct histories of the two countries, and the need to examine more generally the relation between war, the state, and social policy.

The importance of war in the formation of social policy is perhaps most strongly stated by Richard Titmuss, in his essay, "War and Social Policy": "The aims and contents of social policy, both in peace and in war, are thus determined – at least to a substantial extent – by how far the cooperation of the masses is essential to the successful prosecution of war" (emphasis added).(3) How does he come to this conclusion, and is it correct? After raising some questions about Titmuss's argument (the most informed and stimulating contribution to the question by a major social policy analyst), I will propose a different approach, and suggest how it might be applied to a comparison of social policy in the United States and Britain in World War II. My primary concern will be with the relation of war to social policy, the state's organized efforts to affect the health and well-being of the populace, rather than with the war's impact on social or political change in general. In later chapters I

6

shall examine the impact of the war on the British and American states' social policy in the areas of nutrition, tuberculosis, and venereal disease. While these three fields have distinctive histories and characteristics of their own, examination in terms of the conceptual framework developed below illuminates them all.

TITMUSS'S ARGUMENT

Titmuss argues that, progressively, war has become total. It once was a game played between rulers, risking a few subjects as pawns while most social life was undisturbed. Now it involves the whole society. Industry, agriculture, even family life are affected. All are shaped and organized as part of a war effort, the consequences of which are felt long before and after any actual fighting. In this progression from limited to total war, Titmuss traces through four stages the state's increasing concern with the quantity and quality of the population:

- with the quantity of troops, leading to census operations
- with the quality, or fitness for service, of recruits
- with the physical health of the whole population, especially of children, the next generation of recruits
- with civilian morale.

These concerns, induced by wars of increasing scale and intensity, have, Titmuss argues, prompted many if not most social policy developments in Britain. Thus the shocking state of health of working-class troops revealed in the Boer War led to the establishment in 1906 of the school medical service, meals for elementary school children, and other services. In World War II the state's survival depended upon the mobilization and support of almost the whole population. The Education Act of 1944, the Beveridge Report, the National Insurance, Family Allowances, and the National Health Service Acts were all "in part an expression of the needs of wartime strategy to fuse and unify the conditions of life of civilians and noncivilians alike."(4) The universalism of the postwar "welfare state" reflected the extent to which the "cooperation of the masses" was essential to military success.

Titmuss bases his conclusions mainly on his and his colleagues' studies of British social policy in World War II and on Stanislav Andreski's theoretical work, Military Organization and Society."(5) He sees World War II as the typical "modern war," the culmination of a historical development from limited to total warfare. Andreski himself assumes no such progression. His key variable is the "military participation ratio" (MPR), defined as the proportion of militarily utilized individuals in the total population. When the MPR is high, the ruling group must win the masses over to support the war, convincing them that they are fighting for themselves. Social inequalities will narrow, while the rulers will also need tight control over the population. Such a war will foster both egalitarian and totalitarian tendencies. When the MPR is low, the masses can be left alone, but a privileged military elite will develop and social inequalities will widen. He does not assume a historical progression from low to high MPR. He shows how MPR may rise or decline with inventions such as the stirrup, the long bow, or gunpowder, which require different kinds of military organization. However, Andreski points out that, with the exception of postrevolutionary France, the major European powers only adopted universal conscription after severe military defeats. The fact that technico-military factors had already made mass armies more effective than professional ones was not enough to lead to adoption of the former. The external pressure of military competition was also necessary.(6) The Russian Revolution showed, among other things, that ruling classes had good cause to resist mass-conscript armies for as long as possible.

Andreski's indicators of MPR include extent of conscription or national service, proportion of GNP going to the military and to war production, and actual or anticipated civilian injuries. World War II certainly involved a high MPR, and it strengthened statist and egalitarian tendencies, especially in Britain where the MPR was substantially higher than in the United States. In both countries, military success required the participation in the war effort of the working class and specially oppressed social groups (women and, in the United States, blacks). In both countries these groups made substantial gains in terms of employment and income distribution, which were not completely reversed in the postwar period.(7) The concept of the military participation ratio, however, must be seen as only one element in a larger explanatory framework. It does not explain why, although the Boer War led to a school meals program in Britain, the U.S. House of Representatives opposed federal assistance to the school meals program in World War II, despite the evidence of malnutrition revealed by the Selective Service examinations.(8) Moreover, World War II was not typical of later wars, such as Korea or Vietnam. More typical of the present period are interimperialist wars fought by proxy (which avoid direct confrontation between major powers) or wars of national liberation (which do not threaten the "mother country"). Korea was arguably a case of the first kind, Vietnam of the second. Be that as it may, the Vietnam War certainly involved a high MPR for the Vietnamese (and produced egalitarian and totalitarian tendencies within that society), but for the United States it involved a low MPR, a small proportion of GNP (or even of the total military budget), and low rates of conscription and civilian injury. It was also a regressive war in terms of its effects on social inequalities and the real living standards of workers.(9)

Titmuss's generalizations about war and social policy are thus based too narrowly on Britain and World War II. They also fail to see war itself as a member of a larger class, namely social crisis. American historians of social policy point to the Great Depression much as the British do to World War II. It too broke down resistance to social and economic planning, strengthened the role of the state, flattened the social pyramid somewhat, and produced the basic legislation of the "welfare state." No one would claim that the social policy of the New Deal is usefully explained as the state's response to an impending major war.* It is necessary to distinguish the specific impact of war, and of different kinds of war, from the impact that any kind of crisis might have on a given social structure. Titmuss's claims for war as the major determinant of social policy are too large. A major crisis, whether war or depression, is likely to lead to a new level of state intervention, which then has independent effects in the economy and society, thereby preventing a return to the earlier status quo.

Titmuss neglected an important element in the explanation of social policy (except in terms of wartime morale), which is the response of the state and ruling groups to pressures from below. The reforms of the last Liberal government in Britain are not adequately explained as belated reactions to the Boer War, or as preparations for World War I. They also reflect the attempt to hold and incorporate the rising labor movement within the political system of competition between two capitalist parties. The Liberals failed in this attempt in Britain, whereas Roosevelt succeeded in holding labor in the Democratic Party and Johnson had similar success with regard to the black movement in the 1960s.(10) The "cooperation of the masses" may become problematic in circumstances other than war. Capitalism is a highly dynamic, competitive system (war being only the most intense and deadly form of this competition). It generates social costs, dislocations, and oppositional movements that force the capitalist class (or sections of it), however reluctantly, to look to the state and its social policy (and/or forces of repression) for solutions.

None of these qualifications of Titmuss's argument should obscure its implicit point: ruling groups in a class society will take steps to benefit the health and welfare of the population (i.e., of subordinate classes and strata) when they face a situation in which the needs or demands of that population can no longer be ignored.

---

*It is true, however, that many leading New Dealers gained their first significant governmental experience in World War I and that that experience shaped their later thinking; also, that the war metaphor played an important part in the rhetoric of the New Deal; and that World War II was of much greater and more lasting significance for the expansion of the U.S. bureaucracy than was the Depression. See William E. Leuchtenberg, "The New Deal and the Analogue of War," pp. 81-143, and Bruce D. Porter, "Parkinson's Law Revisited: War and the Growth of Government," pp. 50-68.

The needs themselves, however pressing, do not guarantee social provision. Henry Sigerist, the medical historian, pointed out that, in ancient Rome, war led to the establishment of extensive and sometimes elaborate institutions for the medical care of soldiers when "it was in the interest of the army to restore the wounded as quickly and as thoroughly as possible."(11) On the other hand, he observes, the lack of war led to the establishment of medical facilities for slaves, since in peacetime there were no prisoners of war to replenish the supply of slaves and "it became profitable to spend money for the restoration of the slaves' health."(12) In either case, the needs of the ruling class, not those of the potential patients, were the determining factor. Unfortunately, Titmuss himself obscures this point as a result of his social-democratic conception of the state.

The state, in this view, represents the collective interest of society, not merely of the ruling class or group in society. While it may be unduly influenced or even controlled by dominant groups, the state is essentially above class conflicts. The state intervenes to redress inequalities, to impose "social discipline," and assure a measure of economic security for all.(13) The social discipline imposed by war and enforced by the state is seen as being a restraint on individual greed in the interests of the collectivity, rather than, say, as the price that capital has to pay for the preservation of a system based upon inequality and exploitation. Titmuss certainly conceives of class differences, but he sees classes as groups based upon and defined by gradations of wealth, income, occupation, and so on. By contrast a Marxist view would see the two main classes of capitalist society, the capitalist and working classes, as defined by their interdependent antagonistic relation to each other and their specific relation to the means of production.(14) For Titmuss, classes are not necessarily in conflict with each other: together they constitute "society," which can function effectively and humanely in its "search for equity" (a recurrent phrase) given sensible and informed legislation.

The mutual collective interests of all classes, of society as a whole, are given form, in this view, by the state. Thus, when talking of the state's response to war, he easily slips into the first person plural: he writes of "our concern for communal fitness" and how it has followed closely upon "our military fortunes." Referring to civilian morale in World War II, he emphasizes that "millions of ordinary people" had to be convinced that "we had something better to offer than had our enemies."(15) How are "we" going to convince "them"? Titmuss cites the famous post-Dunkirk editorial in The Times, a call for social justice, which reveals the consciousness, unevenly shared in the British ruling class circles to whom the newspaper is addressed, that if "we" are to convince "them" to continue the fighting and the sacrifice, "we" are going to have to make substantial concessions. The significance of Dunkirk for the timing of this editorial, however, is not that this near-disaster led to a great upsurge of cross-class national solidarity, but that, on the contrary, morale among both civilians and troops was then in a precarious state.(16) As Arthur Marwick observes with regard to the blitz: "The expressions of exultation and of social solidarity are to be found almost exclusively in the diaries and comments of middle- and upper-class people. . . . The expressions of hostility to an established system which had failed to provide adequate protection and post-raid services, are to be found among the working class, and also among the more socially conscious of their betters."(17) World War I had ended, in many countries, in strikes, demonstrations, and revolution. This fact was not lost on Britain's rulers in World War II. As Quintin Hogg put it in the parliamentary debate on the Beveridge Report (February 17, 1943): "If you do not give the people reform, they are going to give you social revolution. Let anyone consider the possibility of a series of dangerous industrial strikes, following the present hostilities, and the effect it would have on our industrial recovery. . . ."(18) Wars often begin by masking the contradictions of a class society with widespread patriotic fervor and solidarity; but if they are at all long or difficult they are bound to expose and sharpen those contradictions.

In the course of this discussion of Titmuss's essay, several questions have emerged: the demands or needs of the subordinate classes, and the extent to which rulers are forced by war (or other circumstances) to respond to them, the need of rulers for a healthy military and work force that supports them, and the relation of the state to different classes. The problem now is to relate these elements in a way that will make it possible to understand more clearly the differential impact of World War II on social policy in the United States and Britain. Since, like Titmuss, I am using "social policy" to refer to certain activities of the state, it is also necessary to define a conception of the state. However, full discussion of the Marxist theory of the state, though it informs the present work, lies beyond its scope.(19) Instead, I shall develop those themes that are most significant for the analysis in later chapters.

CLASS, THE STATE, AND SOCIAL POLICY

Social policy in an advanced capitalist society reflects the need of capital for a work force with an adequate level of health, education, and economic and social security (adequacy being a matter of the level of development of the productive forces). The nature of capital (in particular the competitive, anarchic drive to augment itself) prevents its meeting this need without state intervention. Labor costs have increasingly been socialized, that is, paid as taxes and delivered in the form of state-provided benefits or services ("social wage"), rather than being met entirely through the paycheck or provided as fringe benefits by individual employers. At the same time, workers have organized to demand not only higher wages, but also higher social benefits. Their demands do not necessarily stop at what would be, from a capitalist perspective, the optimum point, the minimum level at which no loss of efficiency occurs and there is no threat to the realization of a surplus* (nor do capital's requirements necessarily coincide with the realizable human needs of the workers). Social policy, as well as repression, may also aim at social order, conditions that allow the accumulation of capital to proceed in a relatively harmonious social and political environment. Thus, it may be directed not only at workers and their families, and those temporarily out of work, but also at those on the margins of the work force or outside it altogether.

Just as workers' pressure for higher wages compels capital to rationalize production and raise productivity, so workers' pressure (exerted through their class organizations – unions and parties – and through strikes, demonstrations, and other actions) for decent health, education, housing, and economic security compels capital to rationalize the provision of these, through the state if necessary. Indeed the processes are not merely analogous, but interrelated. Wage pressure induces technological innovation to maintain competitiveness, and these new conditions in turn require a more reliable, healthy, educated work force. Measures are needed to deal with the social dislocations carried in the wake of rapid technological change. From this perspective, social policy may be seen as an "unstable equilibrium of compromise," in Nicos Poulantzas's phrase.(20) The nature and content of the compromise depend – as does the question of what combination of concession and rationalization it involves – on the balance of class forces at a particular conjuncture. Such an equilibrium in no way implies equivalence of power, still less, equal participation in the actual policy-making process.

The locus of this equilibrium is the state, and the state's social policy crystallizes that compromise. The more threatened the capitalist class, in general, the less able it is to solve its problems by "voluntary" means, and the stronger the role the state has to play. Major wars and depressions are crises in which the state is forced to assert its authority against the prerogatives of individual capitals, and the capitalist class is forced to submit, or both may perish. Such crises impose new needs on capital and the state and at the same time render them more susceptible to pressure from below.†

---

*Ira Katznelson has called this point the "social democratic minimum." The function of policy analysis, in his view, is to identify it (Katznelson, "Considerations on Social Democracy," pp. 77-99).

†This does not imply that state organs are independent of and above specific interests and pressures in times of crisis. On the contrary, there is likely to be an accelerated corporatist trend, a partial

The state, in this conception, carries out certain economic and political functions that protect the general and long-run interests of a national capitalist class. In the case of social policy, or the "welfare state," these are essentially to ensure the reproduction of efficient labor power and to maintain social order and harmony.(21) Social policy thus has an economic efficiency function, which contributes to the accumulation of capital through modifying the reproduction of labor power, and a social control function, which contributes to the general reproduction and legitimation of capitalist social relations.*

The exigencies of international competition, economic and military, may impose severe limits on the state's room to maneuver in carrying out these functions, at the same time enforcing them on the state as inescapable systemic requirements. But there is no guarantee that the state will be able either to formulate or to implement the specific policies that would optimally meet the requirements of both economic efficiency and social control. Many obstacles stand in the way of such a comfortable fit of functional requirements and concrete programs.

One of the greatest obstacles to the achievement of a social policy that is rational in capitalist terms is the capitalist class itself. Just as capitalism, in contrast to slavery or feudalism, depends on the functioning of the market rather than political coercion for the extraction of a surplus, so the capitalist, qua capitalist, is concerned with the economic business of making a profit rather than with running the state. A necessary evil, the state confronts the individual capitalist as an alien force, a parasitic drain on the sources of accumulation (surplus value), interfering and overbearing in its regulations and controls. Even where regulations, such as those aimed at occupational safety, or at limiting child labor, may be in the long-run interests of the national capital as a whole (through contributing to the reproduction of an efficient labor force), individual capitalists may have an interest in breaking the law in order to gain a competitive edge on their rivals.(22)

---

integration of employers and trade union bureaucrats into parts of the state machinery. This constitutes a partial negation of the separation of the political and the economic that, in principle, characterizes capitalism (a negation that nevertheless takes place on the basis of that separation, just as "monopoly" develops on the basis of competition and only partially negates it).

*The "economic efficiency" function may be further divided into "social consumption" (or "social wage"), which is part of the capital costs of reproducing labor power, and "social investment" (e.g., some education spending), which raises its productivity. The "social control" function may be (but generally has not been) divided into legitimation and coercion, the latter being for classic Marxist theory the central and defining characteristic of any state.

The mutually antagonistic, competitive, character of the capitalist class, riven with internal divisions and conflicts, not only necessitates a separate institution, the state, with the function of ensuring the political, social, and even economic conditions in which accumulation can proceed. It also guarantees that the state will be subjected to the pressures and resistances of particular segments of capital, or even capitalists in general, in the pursuit of sectional or short-term interests. Such pressures and resistances shape the formation as well as the implementation of policy. Capital, furthermore, is by its nature international, and tends to subvert the plans of particular capitalist states, for example, in its search for cheap or unregulated labor power.(23)

The state, then, in order to ensure the general and long-run interests of the national capitalist class (as against particular and short-run interests and as against the supranational character of capital itself), must be relatively autonomous in relation to it. It must, indeed, be able to enforce its solutions against capitalist resistance, the more so, I shall argue, the more pressing the problem. At the same time, the state needs that autonomy in order to maintain its legitimacy as the principle of unity of the whole nation (the representative, so to speak, of all citizens and not simply of a particular class).

But, as Poulantzas puts it, the "relative autonomy of the state does not imply a coherent and rational will on the part of the agents of the state, as an intrinsic entity; it exists concretely as the contradictory 'play' within the state apparatuses, or even as the resultant of the balance of forces which is condensed in the state."(24) On the one hand, then, the state expresses in its own structures and policies the contradictions and class struggles of the social formation whose unity and cohesion it represents — it is the "condensation of a balance of class forces."(25) On the other hand, the state is constrained by the logic and requirements of capitalist accumulation in a competitive, anarchic world system punctuated by crises of various kinds. But a crisis necessitates an increased coherence and rationality, an assertion of the state's authority even against the dominant class. The problem of achieving the necessary rationality is in part one of articulating the various demands made by different sections of the dominant class and in part one of responding to external threats (from foreign capitals and their armies) and internal pressures from subordinate classes. These "constraints" on policy formation do not necessarily point in the same direction.

The capacity of different states to encroach on the prerogatives of individual capitals, or the (national) capitalist class as a whole, varies widely and limits the possibility of "rational" policy. It is in this sense that I discuss the relative "weakness" or "strength" of the British and American states, that is, in terms of their comparative ability to assert their autonomy and authority. The extent to which the crisis of World War II imposed on these states an objective need for coherence and rationality, and the extent to which each state was able to achieve them, are important historical questions for the present study. In general, the extent of a state's autonomy vis-a-vis the constituent classes of the society, and the extent of the executive's autonomy within the state, seem to be inversely related to the strength and security of the national capitalist class. The tendency to state autonomization in this double sense (the executive vis-a-vis the state system as a whole, and the state vis-a-vis the rest of society)(26) is mainly a result of succeeding crises, combined with a "ratchet" effect, which prevents a return to precrisis "normalcy." For both Britain and the United States, the most important crises in this respect have been wars, above all World War II.

The difficulty of arriving at a rational policy is compounded by the conflict between the various functions of the state, in particular, the conflict that has most often been discussed in terms of accumulation or efficiency versus legitimacy. As James O'Connor puts it in The Fiscal Crisis of the State, "a state that ignores the necessity of assisting the process of capital accumulation risks drying up the sources of its own power, the economy's surplus production capacity and the taxes drawn from this surplus production capacity (and other forms of capital)."(27) Conversely, he argues, a state that openly uses its coercive power to help one class accumulate capital at the expense of others loses its legitimacy. Similarly, others see a contradiction between the state's need both to promote the "common and long-term interest of capital as a whole" (the "efficiency" function) and to secure the support of noncapitalist classes (the "legitimation" function).(28)

The more the state intervenes in the economic sphere, through nationalization, planning, regulation, subsidy, and so forth – that is, the more directly and overtly the state is bound to the accumulation process – the more serious become the problems of legitimation, for the state as a factor of social cohesion and for the market as an institution beyond politics.

The problem of legitimacy arises because as decisions are transferred from the private to the public sphere, from the market to the "public household" (as Daniel Bell, with admitted ideological intent, calls the state sector),(29) they become open and political, matters of conscious, social, and controversial choice. The state sector may supersede areas of private (or corporate) decision making, among other reasons, in order to reduce conflict. However, the effect may be to politicize the conflict rather than to mitigate it. As opponents of capitalism like O'Connor and supporters like Bell have pointed out, this increasing politicization of the economy holds dangers for the system, both in terms of generating unmeetable demands and of undermining the legitimacy of the market and the state. The worker's standard of living depends increasingly not only on take-home pay and fringe benefits, but also on goods and services provided by the state (the "social wage").(30) As it does so, the reformist barriers (imposed by the structure of capitalism) between the economic and the political, between struggles over wages and conditions on one hand and political power on the other, tend to give way. Defense of living standards increasingly depends upon a struggle over social policy, over what proportion of the total social product should go to what purposes and who should decide — precisely the questions that the "free market" eliminates from the political domain.

But planning at the national level does not "abolish" the market any more than planning at the level of the firm. The competitive drive to accumulate capital is no less compulsive, and no less the central dynamic of the system, for being increasingly international in form, or for involving the state. Competition has not become subordinate to political decision making, but rather the reverse. Governments are more and more held responsible for the functioning of the economy (that is, their legitimacy depends in increasing part on their handling of the accumulation task), but subject as they are to the pressures of international competition, they have less and less freedom of action. While the economy has been politicized, the state has in turn been increasingly subject to the exigencies imposed by the economy. The state is subordinated to the economy, not, of course, in the sense that it is a tool in the hands of the corporations, but in the sense that the contradictory process of capital accumulation imposes necessities and limits on the state's activity.

World War II involved, at one level, the pitting of national economies against one another. Production was at a premium and in each country the state organized and disciplined the economy. It went far toward defining what should be produced, in what quantities, and to what uses it should be allocated. These were political decisions, but the state's room to maneuver was severely limited by the intensity and deadliness of the international competition. The war, in fact, gave special urgency both to the efficiency or accumulation function of the state and at the same time to its legitimation function: since manpower was desperately scarce, the military effort depended upon mass conscript armies, and civilian as well as military morale was of vital importance. The state's attempts to resolve the dilemma, to meet the demands imposed upon it by the economic-military situation while maintaining its legitimacy as unifier of the nation, form a major theme of this inquiry. However, there was no simple tradeoff between efficiency and legitimation comparable to the economic division of the national product between accumulation and consumption. Legitimacy depended in part on the efficiency of the state's prosecution of the war (as Trotsky also shows in diagnosing the collapse first of Tsarist authority, and then of the Provisional Government, in the

Russia of 1917).(31) Efforts to control inflation by restricting immediate consumption were themselves largely motivated by the fear of working-class militancy and political disruption in the face of wartime price increases. In partly socializing consumption, however, through "welfare state" programs, rationing, and other controls, the state always faced potential criticism over the equity of its decisions and conflict between its role as organizer of the war effort (accumulation/efficiency) and as a factor of cohesion and national unity (legitimation). This is nowhere more clearly seen than in the British income-maintenance program for the tuberculous, discussed in Chapter 6.

SOCIAL POLICY AND HEALTH IN WORLD WAR II

On the basis of the foregoing discussion, then, it is possible to see World War II as a crisis, which, like the Depression, threatened (or made vulnerable) the national capitalist classes and necessitated the emergence of a "strong state" capable of encroaching on the prerogatives of individual capitalists and overcoming their suspicion and hostility toward it. The "threat," or vulnerability, in the case of World War II, may be seen as in part internal, taking the form of a heavy dependence on the active support of, and participation in the war effort by subordinate classes and strata. This vulnerability to pressure from below (which can be partially offset by suppression of dissent and tight control over the population, but is not fully relieved even by very high levels of repression) is present in any war where there is a high military participation ratio (MPR). In the case of World War II, however, "military participation" must be understood in a broader sense, for it involved a particularly high level of integration of the productive forces and the armed forces.(32) The technico-military demands of this total war imposed on the state the need to subordinate the entire economic life of the country to the war effort, and therefore to determine what would be produced, by whom, and often for whom. Planning and controls over many aspects of economic and social life were raised to new levels.

What were the results for social policy? Perhaps the earliest and most urgent area of need to be identified by the state in both Britain and the United States was that of health. As war has become more technological, armies have raised the standards of health for their soldiers. Health standards have been significantly higher for the military than for industrial production, as draft rejection rates have dramatically revealed. In wartime, however, the health of workers (especially those with skills needed for essential production) becomes much more important than at other times (including, of course, a depression) due to the shortage of labor — and the situation is exacerbated by measures taken to meet the health needs of the military.

The medical rejection of 40 percent of the first million men examined for military service in the United States caused considerable alarm, especially in view of the low minimum requirements, the army's expectation of only a 20 percent rejection rate, and the fact that those examined presumably constituted the healthiest part of the population.(33) The Selective Service examinations revealed, among other things, serious problems of malnutrition, a fact widely publicized by the National Nutrition Conference for Defense (May 1941) and by Senator Claude Pepper's Subcommittee on Wartime Health and Education. Attention was also focused, both in social policy and business journals, on the tremendous loss to industrial production (running at about 400-million "man days" annually) due to illness.(34)

The war, then, exposed these and other health problems or, more accurately, made them a problem for the state. It also aggravated the situation. The entry of physicians and nurses into the armed forces exacerbated shortages and maldistribution of health care professionals and services in the civilian sector. By 1943, there was one physician for every 100 American servicemen, but only one for every 3,500 civilians. The poorer rural areas of the country with the greatest shortages often overfilled their quotas of physicians for the military, while more urban and prosperous areas failed to meet theirs, thereby increasing the maldistribution. The physicians who continued to tend civilians were likely to be older or in poorer health than those in the army. The situation was especially bad in the war-boom towns, where thousands lived and worked in dangerous, crowded, and unsanitary conditions.(35)

In spite of these problems, the war produced a substantial improvement in health status and health care in almost all fields, whether measured by public and private expenditures, hospital beds, number of physicians and other health personnel, life expectancy, infant mortality, or incidence of most diseases.(36) Much of this improvement was, of course, an unintended side effect of the war, derived from the general improvement in the living standards of the population as labor scarcity (gradually and unevenly) replaced mass unemployment. People could afford to eat better and to spend more on health care – and they did both. In part, however, it reflected the conscious recognition, within the state and among business leaders, that the national health had become a matter of grave importance, to an extent it had not been in the previous decade.

Such was the difficulty of attracting and retaining an adequate work force that employers' concern with their workers' health reached new levels and found expression in many ways, from handing out vitamin pills, to providing physical examinations, hot meals, improved health and safety conditions (especially where women were employed), and, most significantly for the long term, involvement in various forms of health insurance. Perhaps the most conscious industrialist in this field was Henry J. Kaiser, who not only saw the importance to production of a healthy work force and supported prepaid medical care for all, but also instituted his own prepaid group medical care scheme (with the assurance of federally guaranteed profits from war contracts) in the face of intense opposition from the American Medical Association.

The state's response to the health problem also took many forms. Some 16 million servicemen and their dependents were provided with a program of socialized medicine, albeit a short-term one. Many preexisting conditions were treated (especially defects of teeth and eyesight) and about 2 million men were salvaged for military service as a result of induction examinations. Many servicemen received good medical treatment and a balanced, adequate diet for the first time in their lives. In the war-boom towns the federal government financed the construction of hospitals and clinics, and in many cases the U.S. Public Health Service provided more and better services than had existed before the war.(37) A long-term effect of the war was a substantially increased government role in health care financing, especially in the fields of hospital construction, research, education, and mental health.

In Britain a similar pattern emerged: 1) serious problems of health, and of health care organization and financing, 2) exigencies of war, which rendered these problems visible and immediate while at the same time aggravating them, and 3) a response by the state and employers (in this case, primarily the state) which, in conjunction with other factors, led to improved health, a rationalization of the health care system, and a substantial increase in the state's role.(38) There are, of course, important differences. These have to be explained within the framework of the differential impact and nature of the war and the different social formations (i.e., the distinct conjunctures of economic, political, ideological, and social elements) upon which the war made its impact.

As Titmuss documents in his Problems of Social Policy, the Emergency Medical Service had very early to recognize that war-time planning must include provision for civilians. A much higher casualty rate for civilians was expected than actually occurred, but civilians still suffered a higher number of casualties than the armed forces until the third year of the war.(39) The special treatment and privileges that soldiers and veterans receive in wars with a low MPR had to be extended to the whole population, culminating in this case in the provision of a universalist National Health Service. Again, as Titmuss shows, the dependence of the war effort on the support and sacrifice of the working class undermined or made intolerable many of the class distinctions and privileges of prewar Britain, and made possible a degree of universalism in social policy in the 1940s from which successive governments of both parties have steadily pulled back.

In the United States the state was less seriously threatened from outside than Britain (the only major European country not to be defeated in the course of the war). It was therefore less dependent upon the enthusiastic support and sacrifice of the whole population. Concessions and benefits, consequently, were directed more selectively at the pressure points, particularly toward the military and skilled and/or organized labor. The military/civilian distinction remained intact (despite a heavier rate of casualties in war industries than in the armed forces)(40) and the substantial gains made by soldiers and veterans, in health, education, and welfare provision, were not extended to the population as a whole. Veterans' benefits were, as Harold Wilensky puts it, a back door that did not in this case open to the rest of the population.(41) As a result of these social policies, World War II veterans became a relatively privileged part of the population.(42) This partiality of provision was, of course, facilitated by a politically weak labor movement, which, despite the trade union gains of the 1930s, had failed to organize an independent labor party. In Britain, on the other hand, the social-democratic ideology of the Labour Party lent itself admirably to the carrying out of a substantial program of capitalist rationalization by the state, which included some real benefits for the working class, under the guise of an advance toward socialism, or at least toward social justice.(43)

The relative weakness of the threats from outside and below in the United States made it possible for the professional monopoly of the American Medical Association to withstand the pressure of organized labor for adequate health care, or rather to divert it into private and localized channels. The conjuncture of AMA opposition to public health insurance, the needs of capital, the pressures of labor, and the interventions of a state at war resulted in a rapid expansion of collectively bargained health coverage for workers.(44) The result was no national health insurance or national health service, but instead an array of fringe benefits, the extent and adequacy of which varied with the bargaining position of the workers involved.

In view of the considerable disparity in the effect of World War II on national social policy, it is not surprising that British and American writers have viewed the relation of war to social policy so differently. These differences no doubt reflect the general neglect of World War II's importance for American social policy developments, but they also reflect real variations of historical experience. I have attempted to develop an approach within which both national experiences can be understood. Based upon a conceptualization of the state as relatively autonomous but neither independent in relation to the balance of class forces and the requirements of capital accumulation nor necessarily a rational and coherent subject, this approach takes account both of the nature of the war and the demands it made upon each state, and also the nature of the societies upon which the war had its impact. Succeeding chapters will examine the nature of the problems with which World War II confronted the British and American states in certain areas of public health policy, and the character of each state's response.

NOTES

(1) Max Lerner, "The State in War Time," in Willard Waller, ed., War in the Twentieth Century, p. 414.

(2) Maurice Bruce, Coming of the Welfare State, p. 326.

(3) Richard M. Titmuss, Essays on "The Welfare State," p. 86.

(4) Ibid., p. 84.

(5) Titmuss, Problems of Social Policy; Sheila Ferguson and Hilde Fitzgerald, Studies in the Social Services; Stanislav Andreski, Military Organization and Society.

(6) Andreski, Military Organization, pp. 68-70.

(7) See, for example, Arthur Marwick, War and Social Change, pp. 159-61, 171-78; Joan Ellen Trey, "Women in the War Economy," pp. 40-57; Valerie Kincade Oppenheimer, Female Labor Force; William F. Chafe, American Woman; Neil Wynn, "Impact of World War II on the American Negro"; Geoffrey Perrett, Days of Sadness, pp. 310-24; Alan S. Milward, Economic Effects of Two World Wars, pp. 31-33.

(8) See Chapter 5, below.

(9) A. Dale Tussing, "Social and Economic Results of the (Vietnam) War," in Max Casper, ed., The War and Social Welfare, Syracuse, N.Y.: Central New York Chapter of National Association of Social Workers, 1971. The Korean War, which took a considerably larger proportion of the GNP, also involved substantially greater gains in real disposable weekly earnings for private nonagricultural workers (Economic Report of the President, Washington, D.C.: Government Printing Office, 1976).

(10) Cf. Leon Trotsky, On the Labor Party in the United States. On the Great Society and the black movement, see Frances Fox Piven and Richard A. Cloward, Regulating the Poor, ch. 9.

(11) Henry E. Sigerist, "War and Medicine," p. 34.

(12) Ibid., p. 341.

(13) Where Andreski talks of the totalitarian tendencies fostered by a high MPR, Titmuss talks of "social discipline," which he treats as a virtue. For a classic discussion of this phenomenon from an antistatist perspective, see Randolph S. Bourne, "The State," in War and the Intellectuals, pp. 65-104.

(14) On these different conceptions of class, see Isaac D. Balbus, "Ruling Elite Theory vs. Marxist Class Analysis."

(15) Titmuss, Essays on "The Welfare State", pp. 81, 82.

(16) William Rankin, "What Dunkirk Spirit?"; Angus Calder, People's War, pp. 136-39.

(17) Marwick, War and Social Change, p. 156.

(18) Hansard, vol. 386, par. 1816.

(19) A fuller discussion is, however, attempted in the dissertation upon which the present work is based: Paul Adams, "Health of the State: British and American Public Health Policies in the Depression and World War II," D.S.W. dissertation, University of California, Berkeley, 1979, pp. 22-87.

(20) Nicos Poulantzas, Political Power and Social Classes, p. 192.

(21) James O'Connor, Fiscal Crisis of the State, pp. 6-8, 40, passim; Ian Gough, Political Economy of the Welfare State, pp. 44-54, 158-61; Paul Adams, "Social Control or Social Wage."

(22) Hal Draper, Karl Marx's Theory of Revolution, vol. 1, ch. 14; David Vogel, "Why Businessmen Distrust Their State"; John Holloway and Sol Picciotto, "Capital, Crisis, and the State," p. 79; Joachim Hirsch, "State Apparatus and Social Reproduction."

(23) Colin Barker, "The State as Capital"; Nigel Harris, Competition and the Corporate Society, pp. 253-54; Colin Crouch, "Varieties of Trade Union Weakness: Organized Labour and Capital Formation in Britain, Germany, and Sweden," pp. 87-88.

(24) Poulantzas, Classes in Contemporary Capitalism, p. 164. See also Holloway and Picciotto, ed., State and Capital, p. 25; Hirsch, "State Apparatus," pp. 100-1.

(25) Poulantzas, Classes, p. 161.

(26) Draper, Karl Marx's Theory, vol. 1, pp. 311-12.

(27) O'Connor, Fiscal Crisis, p. 6.

(28) See, for example, Claus Offe, "Introduction to Part III: Legitimacy Versus Efficiency," in Leon N. Lindberg et al., eds., Stress and Contradiction in Modern Capitalism, pp. 245-59. For an analysis based on the idea of a contradiction between accumulation and legitimation, see Alan Wolfe, Limits of Legitimacy.

(29) Bell, "The Public Household — On 'Fiscal Sociology' and the Liberal Society."

(30) Adams, "Social Control," pp. 48-51.

(31) See, for example, Trotsky, History of Russian Revolution, vol. 1, p. 382. Cf. Arthur L. Stinchcombe, Theoretical Methods in Social History, pp. 34-37.

(32) Hans Speier, "Class Structure and Total War"; idem, "The Effect of War on the Social Order."

(33) Perrett, Days of Sadness, p. 330. Cf. U.S. Federal Security Agency, Proceedings of the National Nutrition Conference, pp. 63-67. See also ch. 5, below. Draft rejection rates were alluded to in almost all contemporary discussions of the nation's health.

(34) Frank G. Boudreau, M.D., "Food for a Vital America," pp. 128-29, 156-57. This article forms part of a special issue of Survey Graphic on health in wartime, "Fitness for Freedom." For evidence of business concern, see "Death on the Working Front," supplement to Fortune, 26, 1 (July 1942).

(35) U.S. Office of War Information, Doctor Shortage and Civilian Health in Wartime. O.W.I. no. 2398 (Sept. 6, 1943), Washing

ton, D.C.: mimeographed; Elin L. Anderson, "Organizing the Community for Health Protection in Wartime," pp. 262-67.

(36) U.S. President's Commission on the Health Needs of the Nation, Building America's Health, Washington, D.C. Cf. Monroe Lerner and Odin W. Anderson, Health Progress in the United States, pp. 20, 33-36, 43-55, passim.

(37) Robert J. Havighurst and H. Gerthon Morgan, Social History of a War-Boom Community.

(38) Harry Eckstein, English Health Service.

(39) Titmuss, Problems of Social Policy, pp. 335-36.

(40) Fred A. Shannon, America's Economic Growth, p. 814.

(41) Wilensky, Welfare State and Equality, pp. 41-42.

(42) Davis R.B. Ross, Preparing for Ulysses, p. 289.

(43) Anthony Giddens, Class Structure of Advanced Societies, p. 64.

(44) Herman M. Somers and Anne R. Somers, Doctors, Patients and Health Insurance, pp. 226-27.

3

FOOD, NUTRITION, AND
THE THREAT OF WAR

An important and complex area in which both British and American states became involved in efforts to protect the national health was that of nutrition. Its importance lay in its centrality for health, for determining levels of energy and stamina as well as resistance to and recovery from disease. Its complexity lay in its inseparable connection with other areas of policy – especially agriculture and food, economics, and income maintenance policy – which had different aims and priorities.

The approach of war confronted each state with the need to take account of a particular set of policy considerations. The threat and the problems, external and internal, were different in each case: Vulnerability to enemy action, to working-class pressure, or to resistance from agricultural interests varied widely. Together with the nature of the state system in each country, these problems defined the character of the policy response, or range of options, open to each national government.

NUTRITION, HEALTH, AND POLICY

Most of the fall in mortality in the past century and a half has been due to a reduction in deaths from infectious diseases. Nutrition has played a central role in this decline, more important, Thomas McKeown argues, than changes in the virulence of the infectious organism or, through natural selection, in the genetically determined resistance of the host.(1) It was more important too than immunization and therapy, which became effective in most cases long after the disease went into decline. Nutrition affects both resistance to infection and the course and outcome of an infectious disease.(2) Even when, before vaccination, almost all children in all countries caught measles, their mortality from the disease varied according to nutritional level. It was 300 times higher in the poorer countries than in the richer ones.(3)

Nutrition, then, is a matter of central importance to a state concerned with the maintenance and protection of health. Of course, this fact may be more or less well understood. It is only recently that protagonists on all sides of the American debate about national health insurance have stopped quoting figures about the population's health status as evidence for or against a particular system of medical care. They have come to recognize that the "Great Equation, Medical Care equals Health," is wrong.(4) Much of the research linking noninfectious disease, such as hypertension, heart disease, and cancer, to such dietary factors as inadequate fiber intake or excessive sugar or salt, is recent and controversial. Most of McKeown's historical research, indicating the supreme importance of nutrition in determining British mortality rates and population trends over the last 200 years, has been published within the last 20 years.

Nevertheless, as the following chapters describe, nutritional research was thriving in the 1930s and its findings were widely disseminated. Nutritional deficiency diseases such as rickets and scurvy were common among the poor, and their relation to diet was well understood. "But," as nutritionists in the 1930s were also aware, "long before pronounced signs of scurvy, rickets, etc., appear, there is a state of subnormal health which shows itself in slow growth, nervous disorders, impaired digestion, and inability to resist the attack of infective disease."(5)

There is no easy step, however, from recognition of the key role of nutrition as a determinant of health to agreement about the policy implications for the state. For if nutrition affects every aspect of health, policy is no less pervasive in its impact on nutrition. Economic, fiscal, and monetary policy, insofar as it affects working-class living standards, necessarily shapes the nutritional status of the population. Income maintenance policy may be more or less successful in limiting malnutrition through increasing the purchasing power of the poor. Agricultural and food policies help determine how much food is avialable to the consumer and at what price. All this remains true even if a government has little or nothing by way of a specific and deliberate policy for nutrition. Nutrition policy has to be distinguished from policy that affects nutrition, and both from other, nonpolicy determinants of nutritional status.

Total war, with its heavy demands on the labor power and loyalty of the population, makes health a concern of the state. But it does not follow that nutrition, despite its importance for health status, will be central to health policy, or even to food policy. In the case of health policy, there is no guarantee that the state's agents will fully integrate existing knowledge about the importance of nutrition into their policymaking. They themselves are likely to be influenced by prevailing medical and other ideologies, which exaggerate the role of medicine in maintaining health. Whether they are or not, their freedom to maneuver, to plan comprehensively, is highly restricted, even in war. As we have seen, the interplay of potentially conflicting goals (such as efficiency and legitimation) and interests (different sections of capital, professional groups, organized labor, and so on) may issue in policy that is less than rational or coherent.

Even when policy has specifically nutritional goals, as in the case of subsidized (and potentially allergenic) milk or orange juice for infants, or the decision to give priority to importing animal fats and sugar, it is arguable that the result is more to undermine than to reinforce nutritional status. In the same way, the use of mass radiography may have done more to promote cancer than it did to control tuberculosis.

Policy that does help may be aimed at something else. This clearly may be the case with economic policy in general, and income maintenance in particular, neither of which is usually seen as a component of public health or nutrition policy. Similarly, both nutrition policy and other policy affecting nutrition may be more important in controlling tuberculosis than all measures taken with that end specifically in view. (Housing policy is also not typically conceived as part of a public health policy to control infectious diseases, but it may have more impact, positive or negative, on the control of tuberculosis than case finding, X-rays, immunization, and therapy.) Finally, it is important to recognize that policy of any kind is of limited efficacy and may be much less important in improving nutrition (or reducing tuberculosis) than the course of economic development and class struggle. Both may proceed in spite of policy aimed at furthering or inhibiting them.

The concern of this study is with the impact of crisis on the state's involvement in efforts to improve or maintain the health status of the population and not, except incidentally, with the effectiveness or appropriateness of those efforts in the light of present public health thinking. In the depressed 1930s, the approach of war called for a redirection of policy with respect to the national food supply and the nutritional needs of the British and American populations. The challenge was different in each case, as was the state system that attempted to meet it.

WAR AND FOOD

Famine is the traditional companion of war. The first concern of a state at war is to avoid being starved into submission. Far short of starvation, however, food shortages and price rises pose a threat to stability and order, which may be serious enough to result in defeat or revolution. Maintaining physical fitness through a nutritionally adequate diet, however much war makes it an official concern, is unlikely to be the first priority of food policy.

Nutritional adequacy, then, has to take its place among other policy goals, such as controlling inflation and forestalling industrial militancy. Food policy itself is but one aspect of a national mobilization that requires a balancing, a series of tradeoffs, between different needs, and a high level of coordination between agencies, departments, and other units within the state system. The U.S. federal government's account of its own war program brings out in this passage some of the complexities involved in trying to articulate food policy with the general management of the war.

> In carrying out a food-production program it was necessary to determine which commodities were most essential to conduct of the war; to persuade millions of farmers to plant essential war crops and to take risks involved in shifting to new crops; to balance the need for imported foodstuffs against requirements for manganese and chrome and to assign shipping space accordingly; to divide the Nation's labor force among farms, factories, and the military services; to decide whether plants should continue to make farm machinery and food processing equipment or convert to production of tanks and guns; and to decide whether chemicals should be used to manufacture antityphus and antimalaria insecticides or refrigerants for food storage facilities.(6)

In developing food plans for the impending war, Britain and the United States faced very different problems in the 1930s. The important differences were not those of nutritional status. The American prewar diet was somewhat higher in calories, and included more dairy products, poultry, eggs, and fruit, but the overall difference in nutritive value was probably small.(7) Contemporary surveys showed great variation in nutritional levels within each country, however, with a large part of both populations subsisting on inadequate diets.(8)

It was in the kind of threat posed to the food supply, and in the capacity of the state to respond coherently and decisively that the important differences between the two countries resided. Britain depended heavily on imports. Its agricultural sector had shrunk dramatically in the half century before World War I, and the decline continued in the interwar years.(9) It was, as the 1914-1918 war had shown, likely to be subjected to enemy blockade aimed at cutting off the food supply. On the other hand, World War I, "a war of competing blockades,"(10) had also demonstrated how, with effective state control, the loss of usual imports could be sustained without the disastrous consequences on which the Germans had counted in developing their submarine strategy. Government control made it possible to use shipping space to the best advantage, while rationing enabled the state to allocate the national food supply with minimal waste. Precisely because so much land had been freed from cultivation in the previous 50 years, there was considerable scope for increasing domestic production by bringing unfarmed land back under the plough. World War I also showed the possibility of substantially increasing the nation's food supply by ploughing pastures and planting them to grain. This shift from livestock to cereals and potatoes also freed scarce shipping space that had been used for importing animal feedstuffs.(11)

All these measures required the positive and effective intervention of the state. The exigencies of war pushed aside the obstacles to a high degree of state autonomy and control. Not the least of these in 1914 was a strong liberal commitment to laissez faire economic principles, an ideology powerful enough to have minimized British preparations for war. Germany, in contrast, had long striven, through tariffs and other means, to escape dependence on foreign food. It produced, before World War I, 80 percent of the calories it consumed, compared with Britain's 35 percent, and had substantially higher productivity per acre.(12)

Put to the test of war, however, Germany proved to be much less flexible in substituting for food lost to bad weather and enemy blockade. The effects on civilian death rates and morale were disastrous and may have been decisive to the outcome of the war.(13) In part, perhaps, the failure was due to a more limited scope for increased agricultural productivity and for bringing new land under cultivation. More significant, however, was the inability of the German state, with a less developed and efficient civil service, to impose effective controls on its more heterogeneous population. Sharper divisions between town and country were especially significant: the state was unable even to persuade German peasants to reduce their numbers of livestock so as to divert cereal production to direct human use. It was equally powerless to impose an equitable distribution of food. "Producers kept all they needed themselves, and more," General von Ludendorff complained, black markets flourished, and the poor went hungry.(14)

Both state system and social structure, then, shaped the differential capacity of Britain and Germany to withstand an effective blockade in the first world war.* "Food," as Sir John (later Lord) Boyd Orr noted in 1940, "was a decisive factor in the last war."(15) As World War II approached, Britain again faced the prospect of a

---

*That the German U-boat campaign was effective may be seen by its surpassing its goal of sinking 600,000 tons of shipping per month between February and August of 1917. The miscalculation was that this would force Britain to make peace. (Olson, Wartime Shortage, p. 83.)

submarine blockade and other threats to its food supplies. It was even more dependent on imports and its agricultural sector had shrunk a further 25 percent or so.(16)

For the United States, the situation was different. American agriculture produced more than its domestic market could absorb and the country's food supplies did not face any serious danger. On the other hand, the task of organizing, rationalizing, and controlling the national food supply was immensely more difficult. The British government could without great difficulty take control of all imports, from purchase to distribution. But the American state would have to deal with a widely dispersed and politically influential agricultural sector. There were several million small producers, many of them operating family farms, who were accustomed to growing certain crops and whose traditional production patterns were enshrined in a jealously guarded "parity" structure developed in the context of economic depression.(17) Control of food distribution required that

> ... provision had to be made for equalizing supplies between the country's producing and consuming areas; procuring food for military services without disruption of local markets and in accordance with seasonal fluctuations of supply; and for moving raw foodstuffs to processors so that luxury commodities were not produced at the expense of necessities or supplies of processed foods were not taken out of the ordinary trade channels.(18)

The British experience in World War I seemed to show that effective control required regulation of every stage of production, distribution, and consumption. But the United States was much more heterogeneous, being divided between urban and rural, industrial and agricultural interests, as well as along regional, ethnic, racial, religious, and other lines, and such a level of control would be difficult to establish even with a strong, highly legitimate, centralized state. However, the American state system was much less centralized and integrated than the British, and less autonomous vis-á-vis particular and sectional capitalist interests. American business was, indeed, so secure internally and internationally, that it was able to enjoy the luxury of antistatism to an exceptional degree.(19) Despite the centralizing impact of the depression and New Deal, the American state remained, by international standards, extraordinarily weak, fragmented, and incoherent. Impending war did not threaten its food supplies as it did the British, but given the character of American society and its state, the task of minimizing waste, ensuring equitable distribution, and providing food for its troops and allies, while controlling inflation, would be formidable.

FOOD AND THE WORKING CLASS

War imposes on the state a double burden with respect to the working class. On the one hand, the task of ensuring the reproduction of labor power for industry and manpower for the military becomes more costly and difficult. Standards of physical fitness for the military are higher than those required for industrial production, and, as labor surplus gives way to scarcity, industrial workers are required to work more intensely but are less easily replaced. Adequate nutrition was, and was seen to be, central to carrying out the task of reproducing the military and work force at a sufficient level of health.

On the other hand, in a war that depends upon mass participation and support, the state requires, much more fully than at other times, collaboration and solidarity between classes. The level of social cohesion, the degree of national unity, that the state must achieve rises with the external threat and the dependence upon subordinate classes and strata. In Britain, faced with the prospect, externally, of German bombing and even invasion and, internally, of an absolute labor shortage, the legitimacy of the state and the morale of the civilian population were especially urgent concerns.

A social policy might aid mass mobilization for total war both by enhancing the physical fitness of the working population and, at the ideological level, by providing an expression of social harmony and solidarity. The importance of food policy in this respect was widely recognized. As the fates of Germany and Russia in World War I seemed to show by negative example, adequacy and equity in the provision of food were shields against defeat from without and revolution within. "I was well aware," J.R. Clynes, British Food Controller in the last part of World War I, wrote of the danger in 1917, "that lack of bread is the root cause of most revolutions, and that this lack could cause one in England just as quickly as it had recently done in Russia, or as it was yet to do in Germany.(20) Clynes recalled in his Memoirs how Lord Rhondda, his predecessor as food controller, had told him: "Without rationing, we're done. It might well be, Clynes, that you and I, at this moment, are all that stand between this country and revolution!"(21) His Memoirs were published in 1937, and this passage was often quoted in the next few years.(22)

A serious revolutionary threat to the state from the working class, however, depends upon a cohesive political organization that institutionalizes the revolutionary purpose and poses it concretely as a socially available strategy. Such an organization, on a scale to make it credible, did not exist in either country. The British labor movement of 1939, unlike the American, had its own mass political party. Firmly reformist and statist in its conception of socialism, bureaucratized in its structure, and with a leadership that was anything but revolutionary, the Labour Party provided a vehicle for directing working-class discontents and aspirations into relatively safe channels.

The defeats and retreats of the previous two decades of more or less severe depression had, moreover, severely weakened the British labor movement. Those years saw wage cuts, reductions in unemployment benefits, layoffs and mass unemployment, punctuated by the crushing defeat of the General Strike in 1926. This was followed by the Trades Disputes Act (which outlawed solidarity or "sympathy" strikes) in 1927 and the political disintegration of the Labour Party leadership and devastating electoral defeat of 1931. Union membership fell sharply after the failure of the General Strike, to less than 5 million in 1927, the first time it had been that low since 1916. It dropped to 4.4 million in 1933, only just above the 1914 level, rising slowly back to 6 million at the start of World War II.(23)

The Labour Party lost five sixths of its parliamentary seats in 1931, being reduced to 46 against the National Government's 556 seats. In 1935, despite a high popular vote, Labour increased its representation only to 154, leaving the Conservative-dominated National Government with a huge majority in a parliament that was highly unrepresentative and would become more so in the ten years that intervened before the next general election.(24)

When war came, the labor movement had been increasing slowly in industrial and political strength, and the working class had experienced slowly rising real incomes despite very high unemployment in certain areas. But both the class and its organized expression in the unions and Labour Party still bore the marks of subjugation, the loss of confidence and narrowing of horizons that follow a major defeat and are only slowly overcome.(25)

There was, therefore, less governmental concern about the likelihood of organized revolutionary opposition than a distrust of the working class's loyalty and morale. Much more damage and loss of life from bombing were expected than actually materialized, and much greater panic and breakdown of civilian morale were anticipated.(26) In its secret planning for this flight and panic, the government looked first to the army and police, and then to civil defense services to maintain morale, while psychiatrists, expecting millions of cases of hysteria and acute neurosis, called for massive expansion of mental health services. In March 1939 the Ministry of Health, upon considering the problem of air raid refugees, asked the India Office to recommend an official experienced in the "management" of large masses of people. The outcome was that the ministry's Relief in Kind Committee acquired the services of a retired inspector-general of police.(27)

In the United States, in contrast to Britain and other European countries, no independent party of labor, based on the unions and commanding the loyalty and support of a majority of the working class, had emerged from the bitter labor wars and the growth of unionism to become the political arm of the labor movement. In the two-party system, both parties remained capitalist, two wings, as Gore Vidal likes to say, of a single Property Party.(28) Despite the tradition of "pure and simple" business unionism represented historically by Samuel Gompers (what C. Wright Mills called a "kind of procapitalist syndicalism from the top"(29)), most of the labor leaders committed themselves to Roosevelt and the New Deal. They looked to the state and the Democratic Party as the vehicles for the realization of labor's political aims and for protection from antilabor forces. State regulation of the capital-labor relation advanced dramatically in response to the crisis of the 1930s. In the face of working-class militancy, including general strikes in Minneapolis, Toledo, and San Francisco in 1934 (all led by socialists or Communists), it was increasingly clear that unionism could not be smashed and had better be regulated so as to bring some order to industrial relations. State regulation of labor relations would continue to advance during the war and afterward, the emphasis shifting from the New Deal aim of seeking "industrial stability and class peace by extending the rights of the unions and limiting the rights of employers to destroy them," toward tighter state controls over the rights of the union and its leadership.(30)

The 1930s were a period of weakness and retreat for the labor movement in Britain, and of catastrophic defeat internationally – Hitler triumphed in Germany, Franco in Spain, while in Russia Stalin destroyed every trace of independent working-class activity and subordinated the international Communist movement to the foreign policy interests of the Russian bureaucracy. In the process he disoriented and isolated the revolutionary left throughout the world. In the United States, however, labor made vital gains. The basic mass production industries were organized with astonishing speed, the right to collective bargaining was recognized and to some extent protected by the state, union membership grew rapidly in a prolonged period of depression and mass unemployment. Even the tiny Trotskyist movement, almost all that was left of the revolutionary tradition of classical Marxism, was stronger and more fully integrated with the working class in the United States than anywhere – it led the "teamster rebellion" in Minneapolis in 1934.(31)

However, with some notable exceptions, such as John L. Lewis, the main CIO leaders became increasingly allied with the liberal wing of the Democratic party. Their statism took the form of more or less uncritical support for Roosevelt and the New Deal, rather than of organizing an independent, reformist labor party. It was corporate-liberal rather than social-democratic. Even Lewis, who was not committed to Roosevelt or the Democrats, was a product of the older business unionism of the AFL, rather than an advocate of independent political organization. Sidney Hillman's and David Dubinsky's American Labor Party (ALP), founded in New York State in 1936, was never a nationwide mass party. As a Marxist commentator put it, their party served "to switch the traditional socialist vote away from their old friend Norman Thomas to their new idol Roosevelt, by making it possible for socialist voters to cast their ballots 'independently' for FDR." Far from posing an independent labor alternative to Roosevelt, in 1940 the ALP provided the margin by which he carried New York state.(32).

In neither country, then, did the organized working class appear to present a serious political threat. Labor leaders would be easily brought into a position of collaborating with the state and capital in support of the war. In Britain, the Labour Party's continuing, and reviving, political importance ensured that it would play a more important role in the wartime government. The danger of failing to ensure an adequate and equitable distribution of food lay not in the threat of a successful revolution, but rather in a debilitating loss of morale and support for the war, in food riots and civilian panic. It was a greater danger for the British state because of its more precarious food supply and its more vulnerable military situation. The relative weakness and fragmentation of the American state, it has been suggested, increased the difficulties of adapting food policy to the demands of war. But the "weak state" itself resulted in part from the historical weakness of the working-class political challenge it had to face (and in part from the relative weakness of external military threats). Labor's continuing lack of organizational, ideological, and political independence (despite the gains of the 1930s) minimized the state's vulnerability to working-class pressure. Because the supply situation was more favorable and the external threat was weaker, the United States could afford to have a less tightly controlling and egalitarian food policy than would be the case for Britain.

CONCLUSION

Nutrition, then, was pervasive both in its impact on the national health and in its interconnections with other areas of policy. In the context of an impending world war, however, the state's immediate concern was with ensuring an adequate food supply, equitably distributed at reasonable prices. Avoidance of shortages and inflation of the kind that had contributed to defeat in Germany and revolution in Russia two decades earlier was the first priority. Fear of industrial unrest had indeed done far more to stimulate comprehensive food planning in Britain in 1917 than concern about nutritive levels and their impact on health.(33)

The task of "ensuring an adequate food supply," however, clearly includes a nutritional aspect; adequacy has the potential of being defined in terms of nutrition. As we shall see in the following two chapters, war itself would push the state in this direction. Decisions about how to allocate shipping space, to ration food supplies among civilians, to monitor and maintain civilian health, would increasingly be referred to their nutritional context.

As Britain and the United States prepared for the possibility of world war in the late 1930s, both states faced formidable but different problems in the sphere of food and nutrition. The military threat to food supplies was a major consideration for British policymakers, whereas for the Americans it scarcely existed. Their central task was to organize, to mobilize a diverse and complex agricultural sector, and to articulate food policy with the rest of the war effort. There was also, of course, a marked difference in the urgency and severity of the crisis that total war posed for each state in the sphere of food and nutrition, as in other areas. The capacity of each state to meet its problems was not a function of differences in the "baseline" nutritional status of its population. The important differences, rather, were those of the state system (level of integration and adaptability to emergencies) and of social formation (balance of class forces).

NOTES

(1)   Thomas McKeown, The Role of Medicine, pp. 45-65; idem, Medicine in Modern Society, pp. 39-58.

(2)   P.M. Newberne and G. Williams, "Nutritional Influences on the Course of Infections"; McKeown, Role of Medicine, pp. 60-63.

(3)   M. Behar, "A Deadly Combination," World Health (February-March, 1974), p. 29.

(4)   Aaron Wildavsky, "Doing Better and Feeling Worse," p. 105. For influential discussions of this theme, see for example, John Powles, "On the Limitations of Modern Medicine" and A.L. Cochrane, Effectiveness and Efficiency.

(5)   Sir William Crawford and H. Broadley, The People's Food, p. 3.

(6)   U.S. President, Bureau of the Budget, The United States at War, p. 330.

(7)   U.S. Department of Agriculture, Food Consumption Levels, Third Report to Combined Food Board, p. 28. The methodology, but not the general conclusions, of three Combined Food Board reports (1944-1946) are criticized by R.J. Hammond, Food, Vol. 1, pp. 386-88. For an earlier comparative study of consumption levels, see International Labour Office, Workers' Nutrition and Social Policy (1936).

(8)   For Britain, see John Boyd Orr, Food, Health and Income; B. Seebohm Rowntree, Poverty and Progress, pp. 172-97; Crawford and Broadley, People's Food, pp. 122-62; G.C.M. M'Gonigle and J. Kirby, Poverty and Public Health. For the United States, see for example, Hazel K. Stiebeling and Esther F. Phipard, Diets of Families of Employed Wage Earners; Stiebeling et al., Family Food Consumption and Dietary Levels; U.S. Department of Labor, Family Expenditures in Selected Cities, 1935-1936. Vol. 2. For a popular summary of these findings, see Stiebeling, Are We Well Fed?

(9)   K.A.H. Murray, Agriculture, p. 39; Mancur Olson, Jr., Economics of the Wartime Shortage, pp. 73, 117.

(10)   James Arthur Salter, Allied Shipping Control, p.1.

(11)   Olson, Wartime Shortage, pp. 73-116.

(12)   Ibid., pp. 74-75.

(13)   Erich von Ludendorff, My War Memories, Vol. 1, pp. 349-55. It was Lloyd George's opinion, too, that "The food question ultimately decided the issue." Cited by Charles Smith, Food in Wartime, p. 3.

(14)   Ibid., p. 351; Olson, Wartime Shortage, pp. 79-81.

(15)   Sir John Boyd Orr, Nutrition in War, p. 3.

(16)   Murray, Agriculture, pp. 38-39; K.G. Fenelon, Britain's Food Supplies, p. 48.

(17)   U.S., President, Bureau of the Budget, United States at War, pp. 338-39.

(18)   Ibid., p. 330.

(19)   David Vogel, "Why Businessmen Distrust Their State," pp. 45-78.

(20)   J.R. Clynes, Memoirs, vol. 1, p. 214.

(21)   Ibid., p. 234.

(22)   See, for example, Charles Smith, Food in Wartime, p. 3.

(23)   Arthur Marwick, Britain in the Century of Total War, pp. 155, 225.

(24) Angus Calder, People's War, p. 27.

(25)   Leon Trotsky, 1905; idem, History of the Russian Revolution, vol. 1, pp. 35-36; Arthur L. Stinchcombe, Theoretical Methods in Social History, p. 38.

(26)   Richard M. Titmuss, Problems of Social Policy, ch. 2; Tom Harrison, Living Through the Blitz, ch. 1.

(27)   Titmuss, Problems, p. 19, n. 2.

(28)   Gore Vidal, Homage to Daniel Shays: Collected Essays 1952-1972, New York: Random House, 1972, pp. 434-44; idem, Matters of Fact and Fiction: Essays 1973-1976, New York: Random House, 1977, p. 268. For discussion of this phenomenon see Werner Sombart, Why is there no Socialism in the United States?; Jerome Karabel, "The Reasons Why"; idem, "The Failure of American Socialism Reconsidered"; Selig Perlman, A Theory of the Labor Movement.

(29)   C. Wright Mills, Power, Politics and People, p. 109. Cf. Rimlinger, Welfare Policy and Industrialization, p. 81; Ronald Radosh, "Corporate Ideology of American Labor Leaders from Gompers to Hillman," in Weinstein and Eakins, ed., For a New America, pp. 125-52.

(30)   Ben Hall, "Labor Policy," p. 165.

(31)   Farrell Dobbs, Teamster Rebellion

(32)   Hall, "Labor Policy," p. 165. Richard Polenberg, War and Society, pp. 206-7.

(33)   See, for example, F.H. Coller, State Trading Adventure, p. 1; Clynes, Memoirs, Vol. 1, pp. 214, 234.

4

WAR AND NUTRITION: BRITAIN

At the high point of British industrialization, in the early nineteenth century, there occurred in certain cities a marked deterioration in standards of nutrition.(1) For some occupational groups, notably hand loom weavers, starvation was a reality. Malnutrition became common, and persisted unevenly despite a general improvement in diet in the course of the nineteenth century. Poor physical standards of the working population, tolerable in peacetime, became a source of concern to the state in time of war. War, indeed, became the test of the nutritional status of the working class and also the chief impetus for efforts at its improvement. Discussing the effects of the decline of diet on the health of the population, the leading nutritional researcher and publicist, Sir John Boyd Orr, noted in 1943:

> By the middle of the nineteenth century, the majority of poor children in industrial towns suffered from one or more of the nutritional diseases, such as rickets or scurvy. The average stature fell. Twice during the nineteenth century the height of recruits for the army had to be reduced, first from five feet six inches to five feet three inches, and then from five feet three inches to five feet. . . .The deterioration in physique became evident when a large number of recruits were medically examined during the Boer War. . . .The medical examination of recruits in the 1914-1918 war again revealed the poor physical condition of the people.(2)

The implications of nutritional status for the effective prosecution of war led to the extension of official concern beyond the armed forces, to children who would provide the next generation of soldiers, and to industrial workers who provided the munitions and materiél on which the war effort depended. Thus, the Boer War provided the stimulus for a school meals program, and World War I produced a big expansion of industrial catering. The latter war, by revealing the extent and strategic significance of our ignorance about food and nutrition, also gave the impetus for a rapid development of experimental research in the following decade.

While the 1930s saw a growth of concern, publicity, and research in the area of nutrition, relatively little was done to improve the nutritional status of the population until World War II. The war made poor nutrition a problem for British capital as a whole, one that could only be resolved by massive state intervention. This expanded state responsibility went beyond preventing the starvation of the destitute, to ensuring the availability of a nutritionally adequate diet for the whole population while allowing for the special needs of certain groups. It created changes in the economy, in consumption patterns and expectations (political and dietary) that outlasted the end of the war. The market reasserted itself, rationing and state controls were phased out, but the state's responsibility for ensuring the adequate feeding of the population remained greater than before the war; it became part of the social definition of the postwar "welfare state."

THE 1930s: CONCERN ABOUT MALNUTRITION

Advances in nutritional knowledge, surveys revealing nutritional deficiencies, and the publicizing of concerns about malnutrition, all characterized the decade prior to World War II. Each reinforced the other as public concern, for example, stimulated by reports of severe malnutrition among families of the unemployed, generated dietary surveys, which deepened the concern by revealing the extent and seriousness of malnutrition.

The impact of all this on the government, however, was minimal. Despite the appointment of an advisory committee on nutrition in 1931, the government's clear intention was to limit its social service spending as much as possible, and certainly not to uncover new areas of need requiring state intervention. The necessity to cut the dole by 10 percent, accepted by the economically orthodox in all the main political parties, precipitated the collapse of the minority Labour government in the same year. Business confidence had to be restored and new investment encouraged, a policy thought to require lower taxes and cuts in public expenditure. The Conservative-dominated National Government, bolstered by a landslide election victory and supported by the weight of Treasury and business opinion, believed that any expansion of the state's responsibility for the health and welfare of its citizens would be an obstacle to economic recovery and thus against the interests of the nation as a whole.

From this perspective, the work of nutritionists like Boyd Orr, who drew attention to the importance of nutrition for health, to the relationship of adequate nutrition to income, and to the need for a government food policy that fostered better nutrition of the whole population, was an embarrassment. The strong tendency of the government and civil service, then, was to play down the evidence presented by nutritionists and social investigators. As an example of this negative attitude before the war, Titmuss tells of the reception in the Ministry of Health of a 1934 report on health standards by three of the most authoritative experts of the day:

This report, written for the Government's Economic Advisory Council by Professor (later Sir Edward) Mellanby, Sir F. Gowland Hopkins and Sir Daniel Hall, stated that the health of the people was in a "deplorable condition," and made a series of recommendations designed, so it was said, to bring about a national food policy. In comments to the Minister of Health it was dismissed by one high official as an "irregular screed and unreliable outburst," and by another high official as "improper, unfair and heavily overdrawn." It was further said that the authors of the report had thought of nothing else since "their 'discovery' of vitamins"; that the facts they quoted concerning the physique and health of Army recruits were fallacious, and that much was being done by local authorities in giving advice to "dole-receivers as to food values."(3)

The Ministry of Health, nevertheless, together with the Medical Research Council, sponsored much of the nutritional research that showed the need for certain vitamins and for milk in preventing deficiency diseases (such as rickets) and in improving the growth rate, and physical and mental efficiency of young children.(4) The prevailing political climate, however, in government and senior civil service, as well as the specific objections of the Treasury, militated against the translation of such findings into implementable policy. Milk consumption, for instance, was little higher than it had been before World War I, or even a century before, despite the new knowledge of its importance for the health of mothers and children. It declined with income and was lowest among the poorest sections of the population, which contained a disproportionate number of children.(5) Even in the first months of the war, when it appeared that wartime price rises might put milk altogether beyond the reach of those most in need of it, the Treasury found "objectionable" the Ministry of Health's suggestion (in December 1939) that a subsidy might be required.(6)

Orr's dietary survey was carried out in 1935 under official auspices, but the report and its author were somewhat embarrassing to the government. Hence, it was not published in the usual way as a White Paper, but instead appeared as an unofficial monograph, Food, Health, and Income, in 1936. Despite the enormous and international influence of this work, it was studiously ignored by the government. The official report of the Advisory Committee on Nutrition, published the following year, does not mention Orr's book by name, but, as Hammond says, "the whole of this report might be taken as an effort to play down his more sensational conclusions."(7) At the same time the Advisory Committee's report admitted that the nation's diet was, on the average, unsatisfactory, comprising too little milk and cheese and too much sugar. The Committee did not elaborate on the inference, underlined by Orr, that the diet of half the nation was, in varying degrees, even worse.

The national diet, together with income and physique, did improve markedly in the first three decades of the twentieth century. It was better (including more fruit and fresh vegetables, butter and eggs) and also cheaper.(8) As a food-importing nation, Britain benefited from the slump in world food prices during the Depression. Orr's study, however, concluded that, despite improvements, "a diet completely adequate for health according to modern standards is reached only at an income level above that of 50 percent of the population."(9) Those with an average weekly income per head of over 45 shillings (£2.25) had a surplus of all dietary elements considered. While inadequate nutrition persisted far above any contemporary poverty levels, the problem became more serious as income declined. A high proportion of the country's children, between a fifth and a quarter, was in the lowest income group, whose diet Orr found to be very seriously deficient.(10)

Other researchers came to similar conclusions. The emphasis on inadequate income, rather than ignorance, as the main cause of malnutrition, was general. Orr's estimate that at least half the population was poorly fed was also made in the same year by two other researchers, G.C.M. M'Gonigle and J. Kirby.(11) Malnutrition, like unemployment and wage cuts, was experienced very unevenly. Unemployment rates ranged from 67 percent in Jarrow to 3 percent in High Wycombe.(12) For those who bore the brunt of the depression, diets were little if at all better than in the nineteenth century. J.C. Drummond (later, in World War II, Sir Jack Drummond, chief scientific adviser to the Ministry of Food) and Anne Wilbraham, commenting on a 1929 report of the Ministry of Health describing the terrible food conditions in the Welsh coalfields, added:

> ...but the same distressing details were true of a thousand other areas in the country. The diets of the poor working people had become almost as bad as they had been in the worst years of Queen Victoria's reign: white bread, mar-

garine, jam, sugar, tea and fried fish. Meat was seldom eaten more than once a week, while fresh vegetables, other than potatoes, were rarely bought. Fresh milk was hardly ever seen.(13)*

Orr's standard of nutritional adequacy was based on a physiological ideal — "a state of well-being such that no improvement can be effected by a change in the diet."(14) Other researchers followed the British Medical Association's 1933 standards, which were based on the minimum level of nutrition necessary to avoid obvious symptoms of deficiency.(15) Their figures showed one third of the population living below this bare subsistence level, an estimate made also by Orr in 1939.(16) Sir William Crawford's investigation, based on an extensive door-to-door survey of dietary habits in 1936-1937, showed that about one third of the population was deficient in calories and protein, and half or more was deficient in vitamins.(17) His study also suggests the force of tradition and ignorance on eating habits, as well as confirming what other surveys revealed, the persistence among poor families of the nineteenth century pattern of first satisfying their hunger with cheap carbohydrate foods, washed down with countless cups of tea, and only then turning, as they could afford, to high protein foods and green vegetables.(18)

Again and again these dietary surveys show severe malnutrition and poverty persisting amid rising standards of living and eating, with wide variation between classes and between regions. Lady Williams's 1934 experiments in the depressed Welsh mining area of the Rhondda Valley underlined the importance of nutrition for maternal and child health. She found that improvements in prenatal care failed to reduce the high infant mortality rate, until food was distributed to expectant mothers, when it fell by 75 percent.(19) In 1935, 62 percent of volunteers, presumably young men in their prime but from backgrounds of unemployment and poverty, fell below the army's rather low standard of physique.(20) The Pilgrim Trust's 1938 survey of the unemployed, Men Without Work, found 44 percent of unemployed families to be below the British Medical Association's bare subsistence level.(21)

Concern about nutrition, then, grew and became more widespread in the years prior to World War II. Where government policy gave expression to this concern, however, it was shaped by the economic conservatism that was prevalent, though not unopposed, in

---

*A careful recent review of the evidence concludes that conditions in the Welsh coalfields were not typical of those faced by the working class as a whole; that nutrition, and other aspects of health, underwent a general improvement despite the Depression. Orr made the same point, but showed that despite these gains much of the population was malnourished (J.M. Winter, "Infant Mortality," pp. 439-62).

all parties, in the civil service, and in industrial and banking circles. It was also influenced by the consideration that <u>on average</u> people were eating better than ever, that the problem of malnutrition was distributed very unevenly in the population as a whole. Both influences, as well as the weight of Poor Law tradition, tended to ensure that state provision in the nutritional sphere was highly selective. It was seen as an aspect of poor relief, rather than, as some reformers urged, a matter of general public health, in which the state's responsibility was comparable to that recognized in the nineteenth century with regard to sanitation. By 1939, for example, health departments were providing milk, cod-liver oil, iron, and vitamin products, at low costs or free, for expectant and lactating mothers and for infants, but only in clear cases of malnutrition.(22) Cheap school meals were provided only for children first proved to be both "necessitous" and "undernourished" — the program reached only 5 percent of elementary school children.(23) The Milk in Schools scheme, on the other hand, which had started in 1934 as a means of disposing of surplus milk, was supplying a third of a pint of milk a day to 50 percent of primary and grant-aided school children, free or below cost. It was not, however, available in the private schools where the children of the business and professional classes were educated. Its point was to help dairy farmers by expanding the effective demand for their product, while at the same time providing some nutritional benefit for school children who might otherwise have been unable to obtain it.(24)

That the growing knowledge and concern about nutrition took the policy form of some additional in-kind poor relief (and agricultural surplus disposal) was a reflection of ruling-class priorities. These measures were clearly inadequate to the task of ensuring a healthy work-force and reserve of unemployed, still less a healthy, mass, conscript army. In a period of peacetime mass unemployment, with a weak and defeated working class, however, other matters seemed more pressing, in particular the need to hold down government spending and increase business confidence. If labor surplus minimized the importance of the state's social wage function (of ensuring the reproduction of the labor force), the organizational and political weakness of the working class at the same time rendered its social control function (of maintaining social harmony) less compelling. As war approached, the need for an adequately fed working and fighting population became increasingly apparent, and urgent. But it took the defeat and evacuation of British forces from Dunkirk, and the heavy bombing of British cities, to bring home fully the vulnerability of the British state and its dependence upon working-class support. Only then was there a major change, seen as a revolution by some contemporaries, in the state's responsibility for the nutritional adequacy of the nation's diet.

WORLD WAR II

Early Conservatism

The British state entered World War II better prepared in terms of food control than it had been for any previous war. The Food (Defence Plans) Department, established in November 1936 and superseded five days after the declaration of war by the Ministry of Food, had set up a structure of complete commodity controls, integrated within a single ministry, which thus, as Eric Roll puts it, "combined a normal civil service hierarchy with a series of state-run trade monopolies."(25) The lesson of World War I in this area was seen as being that control of any food had been successful in proportion to its completeness.(26) Extensive food control, including consumer rationing, was planned to begin immediately upon outbreak of war. Even the ration books were printed in advance.

Despite its plans to intervene strongly and immediately, the Ministry of Food was at first essentially conservative in its approach to food control, certainly by contrast with the policies it was to be drawn into by the process of war itself. From its beginning, the Food (Defence Plans) Department had been deprived of the staff and the mandate for comprehensive policy development that Sir William Beveridge sought for it. As former official head of the first Ministry of Food, and author of the study British Food Control, Beveridge had been consulted by the Committee of Imperial Defence in April 1936. He was invited to head the new food department, but negotiations with him quickly broke down, ostensibly over financial matters, but probably over fundamental disagreement with the transdepartmental comprehensiveness of his approach to civilian war preparations.(27) By the time of the Munich crisis, 21 months after the food department's inception, little had been done: no commodity control or consumer rationing was ready to function. Only as war became more imminent, and the lack of preparedness more evident, did the size and scope of the department and the pace of its activities change.

Even after war had been declared, Ministry of Food officials saw their task as having nothing specifically to do with nutrition. As Hammond puts it, "British food control, as it came into existence at the outbreak of the war, was in no way an instrument for promoting better feeding among the people."(28) It was concerned with inflation, which it saw as resulting from "profiteering." It would procure the "principal" foods and supervise their distribution. It would also control prices, but only insofar as they resulted from profiteering. (Subsidies to offset price rises due to cost increases, although used in World War I and recommended by Beveridge in 1936, were not endorsed by the government of the day.)

It would see that everyone could get a fair share, which in most circumstances was defined as an equal share, of these foods at a fair price – provided he could pay for it. There its responsibility would end; it would not seek to ensure that the whole population was fed adequately by scientific standards; it would not set out, for instance, to prevent rises in prices that were consequent upon increases in production costs; it would not undertake to organize measures of communal feeding. Officials saw themselves, not as social innovators, but as conservators, aiming to assure that, so far as possible, the existing system of food distribution functioned under war conditions, and intervening only to save it from collapse.(29)

Pressures for Change

All that would change. World War II produced, in the words of R.J. Hammond, the author quoted above who was one of its official historians, "a revolution in the attitude of the British state towards the feeding of its citizens."(30) Not only was food control extended in comprehensiveness under pressure of war, but nutritional criteria also became increasingly prominent in shaping policy. Welfare food programs, some of them developed in the 1930s in a situation of mass unemployment and world food surplus, were expanded in a universalist direction in a situation of full employment and food shortage. In addition to such milk, school meals, and vitamin schemes, other programs were aimed beyond "vulnerable" groups to the population as a whole, especially the work-force. Bread, flour, and margarine were enriched; communal meals, factory canteens, and municipal "British Restaurants" were developed or expanded to provide nutritious food for workers on or near the job, while giving a measure of flexibility to the rationing system. Production of carrots and green vegetables was increased for nutritional reasons, to maintain or increase the supply of vitamins A and C while offsetting the reduction of fruit imports. A Dig for Victory campaign, yielding some 2 or 3 million tons of home-grown vegetables, was launched.

What brought about this dramatic change of attitude and policy? Undoubtedly certain individuals played major roles. One of these was Professor J.C. Drummond, the biochemist and student of the history of diet, who was transferred from the University of London to become temporary scientific adviser to the Ministry of Food in February, 1940. John Burnett goes so far as to say that "the 'welfare' aspects of rationing were largely the product of Drummond's fertile imagination and powers of persuasion."(31) His contribution was to apply the most current nutritional knowledge to the task of planning the nation's food supplies in wartime. He surveyed the nutritional requirements of the population, identified weaknesses (in the area of "protective foods"), and made recommendations for planning imports, home production, and food enrichment to meet the anticipated needs.(32) His position and particular knowledge and skills enabled him to survey dietary needs and deficiencies of the population as well as the overall food supply, and to translate the findings of nutritional science into specific policy terms. He was able to succeed, where Beveridge had failed in 1936, in getting the civil service to look broadly and comprehensively at food policy. Unlike Beveridge, he was also highly knowledgeable about nutrition and creative about the possibility for integrating nutritional goals into overall food control. He interpreted the state's task as going beyond ensuring a food supply for the population, to ensuring that all would receive a nutritionally adequate diet, so that no one's health need suffer because of nutritional deficiency.

Sir John Boyd Orr was one of several other leading nutritionists who were drawn into government service. His 1936 study, Food, Health, and Income, together with other reports from the Rowett Institute, which Orr had founded in 1929, became part of the basis for planning the rationing system. Orr himself was appointed a member of the Cabinet's scientific committee on food policy.

There were certainly problems of coordination and differences of perspective between scientists and bureaucrats, and also between different divisions of the Ministry of Food, especially in the first 18 months of the war. The nutritionists, whom the practical administrators tended to dismiss as unrealistic academicians, could not have been as effective as they were without strong support at higher levels. In the early stages of the war, prior to the formation of Churchill's coalition government in May 1940, Walter Elliott played an important role as Minister of Health. He was medically trained and well acquainted with Orr and other leading nutritionists. He brought them into consultation and was infected with their view that "the war presented a golden opportunity for actually improving the national diet."(33) He intervened with the Ministry of Food to ensure attention to nutritional aspects of food control, and sponsored the National Milk Scheme, discussed below. This scheme was not implemented until after his departure from the government, but it was taken up enthusiastically by Lord Woolton, who became Minister of Food in March 1940, and stayed on under the coalition government.(34)

Lord Woolton was a philanthropic businessman and former social worker. He had a deep interest in nutrition, stemming from his experience in a settlement house in the Liverpool slums, where his next-door neighbor had died of starvation.(35) He conveyed his preoccupation both to the general public and government as a whole through his flair for public relations and use of the media, and to his own top officials.(36)

Personal influences were, then, of great importance in the development of a comprehensive nutrition policy, especially in the early months of the war. One must still ask, however, why were

Drummond and Orr, whose work was downplayed in the 1930s, taken seriously now? Why were the Ministers of Health and Food given authority to work out a national milk scheme, a program long opposed by the Treasury as inflationary and unnecessary?

Several factors converged to ensure that politicians and civil servants came to regard nutrition with a new seriousness. World War II presented the British state with a major external threat, and at the same time made it more vulnerable to pressures from below. The food supply itself was directly endangered by enemy action. With shipping at a premium and supply lines cut or at risk, nutritional value relative to bulk became the key criterion for deciding what foods to import. A healthy work force and military were essential to the successful prosecution of the war, and no government, made conscious of this by an acute manpower shortage, could afford to ignore the evidence of nutritional deficiencies and their contribution to sickness and disability. The medical examinations for the military underlined the point, while health indexes for 1940 and 1941 suggested that the war itself was making matters worse.(37) Not only the health of the working class (on whom the war effort largely depended), but also its loyalty and support were necessary for the waging of this total war. That point was brought home by Dunkirk and the heavy air raids on London and the provincial cities.

In a country heavily dependent upon imports — two thirds of the total food supply came from abroad, including 88 percent of its wheat, 91 percent of its butter, and well over half its meat — less than half the prewar amount of food was being imported by 1942.(38) The German conquest of Europe, and Italy's entry into the war, had cut off major sources of butter, bacon, onions, and tomatoes.(39) Japanese victories in the Far East cut off a large part of Britain's supplies of rice, sugar, tea, and other foods.(40) In this beleaguered situation, agriculture and food policy assumed an economic and strategic importance almost as high as arms manufacture.(41) Every aspect of the feeding of the population, from the growing and importing of food to its sale in stores and restaurants, became a matter of government organization and control. The allocation of the food resources of the entire nation became less a matter of individual and corporate preferences registered in the market and more a matter of the state's social policy decision making.

The government implemented its food policies through a complex and diversified rationing system, subsidies to producers, and maximum price orders. It became the sole importer of basic foodstuffs (while banning the import of luxury foods), and was the sole purchaser of fatstock and milk. Although some foods remained unrationed throughout the war, most were controlled in some way, and Calder does not exaggerate in claiming of the Ministry of Food that

With varying degrees of directness, sometimes through newly created autonomous wartime combinations of formerly independent manufacturers or wholesalers (of which MARCOM produced margarine, and BINDAL distributed imported bacon, but BACAL, confusingly, dealt with butter and cheese), the Ministry controlled the manufacture and distribution of virtually all foods.(42)

The very comprehensiveness of the state's control over food, together with the pressure on imports and on shipping space, pushed it in the direction of applying nutritional criteria to its decisions. Bureaucrats who managed the "public household," to use Daniel Bell's term, had to make collective decisions analogous to those made by managers of private households: given a very limited budget, what foods shall we buy, in what quantities, and how shall we distribute them, to ensure a balanced, adequate diet for all family members? Of course, such decisions are not made solely on nutritional grounds in any household – tea, for example, continued to be procured despite its lack of nutritive worth. As discussed below, food subsidies were motivated by the need to control inflation and the extraction rate of flour was raised to 85 percent in order to save shipping, although it also made the flour more nutritious.(43) Nevertheless, however much permanent civil servants may have disliked the nutritional enthusiasts who had joined their departments, they were pushed by the war itself into taking full responsibility for procuring, organizing, distributing the nation's food and, therefore, for the nation's diet.

The responsibility was especially heavy in view of the vital importance, in this total war, of maintaining the health and morale of the mass of the population. Britain faced an acute labor shortage, and the health of the population therefore became, as it had not been in the 1930s, a matter of direct and strategic concern to the state.

Although there had been fears that the war would reveal and exacerbate the poor health of the population, it appeared at first that there was little cause for alarm. The Minister of Health claimed that only 2.3 percent of men aged 20 and 21 years examined under the Military Training Act were definitely unfit for service. Both military and civilian leaders were pleasantly surprised at these "striking results" (as the Minister called them), and The Times proclaimed the British "An A1 People."(44)

This early optimism proved unfounded. The medical examinations for the military during the early months of the war were so perfunctory that many men who had been accepted were later found unfit for military service. Fears about the nation's health increased as major health indexes, including infant and child mortality, and tuberculosis (where the pattern for the years 1939-1941 closely and alarmingly resembled that of the years 1914-1916), revealed a deterioration in the population's health in 1940 and 1941, a trend that was to be reversed from 1942 on.(45)

The new alarm about the nation's health not only drew the state into an active nutritional policy. Led by the Ministries of Food and Health, and the Medical Research Council, it also stimulated further and closer monitoring, in the form of a large number of investigations and surveys of diet and nutritional status, including vitamin deficiency tests and studies of body height and weight changes. Some of the studies were misconceived or of poor quality, but they illustrate the state's concern in this period about nutritional adequacy and its importance for health.(46) In undertaking to organize and control the feeding of the population, the state, as we have seen, necessarily took upon itself responsibility for nutrition. The numerous studies reflect, even in their haste and misdirection, an uneasy consciousness of this responsibility. They were an expression of "the tendency to play for safety in supplies whenever there was the slightest reason to apprehend the development of dietary deficiency," as Hammond puts it.(47)

"Morale," the vaguely defined concept of the time, was as important as physical health. The government and bureaucracy were concerned from the beginning, both to build morale through propaganda, and to monitor it through surveys of public opinion such as those commissioned from Mass Observation, an opinion-sampling organization, and reported secretly to the Ministry of Information. Early official fears were exaggerated, but morale continued to be a source of concern at the highest levels of government.(48) The importance of a sustaining ideology of social solidarity and universalism was at no time more keenly felt than in the period between June 1940, immediately following the evacuation from Dunkirk, and the temporary suspension of the German bombing of British cities in May 1941. This period, in which the German threat was most serious, marked a qualitative shift in the state's involvement in all aspects of the nation's feeding. In these months the school meals and milk programs lost their poor relief character, a universalist national milk scheme developed to provide milk to all pregnant and lactating mothers and young children, and the resistance to an active, deliberate nutritional policy collapsed at the Ministry of Food and even at the Treasury.

Feeding the Work Force

Communal feeding was, in various forms, organized, financed, required, or encouraged by the government. Special communal feeding arrangements were made for shelters from air raids and for their homeless victims, and for evacuated mothers, while the school meals program was greatly expanded. Several programs were directed at the work force. Their development reflects the great importance attached to maintaining the health and working capacity of those who comprised the very scarce labor supply. It may also be seen as a response to the renewed militancy of workers who, in the midst of a total war and against the combined opposition of the state, the union bureaucracies, and the established political leadership of their class, vigorously defended and used the strike weapon. They set a new British record in 1944, when 3.7 million working days were lost in 2,194 strikes.*

The Ministry of Food provided for the establishment of cheap, nonprofit cafeterias, called British Restaurants, run by local authorities but guaranteed against loss by the Ministry. Like the National Kitchens of World War I, they were originally proposed as a measure of assistance to the poor, who had been hit by the rise of food prices in 1939-1940. They were also advocated as a valuable resource in air raids, which they proved to be. But they came to be thought of as having much wider application than as a form of relief. Many saw them as a way of sustaining and improving the diet of the working class at minimum cost. As Lord Woolton wrote in a letter to civic heads in November 1940, urging the establishment of communal feeding centers, "If every man, woman, and child could be sure of obtaining at least one hot, nourishing meal a day, at a price all could afford, we should be sure of the nation's health and strength during the war . . . ."(49) Their scope never matched such ambitions. They

---

*As in the United States, the most serious challenge came from the coalminers: Kent colliers defied the law, courts, prison and fines — and won. In general, strikes were more frequent and involved more workers than in the 1930s, but they were also shorter and more localized. They were more likely to be over wages and conditions than over union recognition or collective bargaining. They reflected a fragmented, localized, and relatively apolitical form of class struggle — a direct, self-reliant shop-floor militancy that did not depend on national union leaders or political parties. The established trade union and political leaders were collaborating with the state and employers in opposing strikes, while no alternative national rank and file leadership was able to develop. Paradoxically, the more "political" rank and file leaders, for example shop stewards who were in or close to the Communist Party (which after the collapse of the Hitler-Stalin pact pursued an extreme class-collaborationist line) were the most hostile to militant activity. Given the highly democratic character of the British shop steward system, however, such local "leaders" were often dragged along behind their fellow workers. (For a good example, see Zelma Katin, Clippie, pp. 80-81; on official union collaboration with employers and state, and unofficial strike activity, see H.M.D. Parker, Manpower; Angus Calder, People's War, pp. 454-61; Alan Milward, War, Economy and Society, pp. 232-44.

reached a peak of 2,160 in September 1943, compared with a talked-of target of 10,000.(50) In addition to legitimating the availability to the affluent of food off the ration at commercial restaurants, however, they did serve the purpose of supplementing the rations of manual workers, and so formed part of a pattern of ersatz differential rationing.

The government's policy, endorsed by the trade union leadership, was "to allow the maximum possible ration to all rather than differential rations to particular categories."(51) Nevertheless, the British Restaurants and other eating places used mainly by manual workers, as well as work-place canteens, received extra allowances of meat, butter, cheese, sugar, and other rationed foods, over and above what was allowed to other restaurants. Furthermore, special arrangements were made for particular categories of workers: for example, extra rations of cheese were allowed for individual workers for whom canteen or public restaurant facilities were not readily available, such as agricultural and forestry workers.

The Ministry of Food differentiated, in the supplies it made available to canteens and restaurants, on the basis of the nature of the work performed. Canteens and restaurants catering to industrial workers were divided into A and B categories, while other restaurants, cafés, and hotels were placed in category C. Category A, catering for workers in heavy industrial jobs such as building, mining, heavy engineering, and shipbuilding, were granted the most generous allowances of rationed food (twice as much meat, for example, as category C). Category B, consisting of all other industrial workers, received somewhat less generous allowances of some rationed foods, but still substantially more than the nonindustrial category C. While this differential provision compensated to some extent for the absence of differential rations for workers in heavy manual occupations, such as were provided in the more complicated German system, it was not so effective in meeting the special needs it recognized. As Calder observes,

> But the canteens were not universal, as a differential ration would have been. Even those which existed rarely had room for all the employees, and transport workers, police, shipyard workers and dockers, all enduring arduous conditions, were still notably short of feeding facilities.(52)

Nevertheless, the scale and extent of the state's involvement in in-plant feeding of industrial workers dwarfed all previous efforts, again reflecting the heavy dependence of the war effort on industrial production and the desperate labor shortage.

Industrial catering can be traced at least to 1618 in England.(53) It developed slowly, however, so that by the beginning of World War I in 1914, there were only about 100 factory canteens. During that war, the government stimulated the rapid development of industrial feeding, both by legislation (e.g., rules issued under the Defence of the Realm Act by the Ministry of Munitions requiring a canteen and the provision of milk where TNT was used), and by encouragement and assistance given on a voluntary basis. By 1918, the Chief Inspector of Factories estimated that there were nearly 1,000 factory canteens in operation or under construction.(54) There were no further compulsory provisions until World War II, but by then the number of industrial canteens had risen to about 1,500.(55)

During World War II a number of Factories (Canteens) Orders were issued by the Ministry of Labour and National Service, requiring the establishment of "suitable" canteens serving hot meals in factories employing over 250 persons, first in munitions and other defense plants (November 1940), then extending to all factories (April 1943). Two other orders, issued in 1941, extended the canteen requirement to cover construction workers engaged in war-related work, and dockworkers. Special provision for coalminers was made, also in 1941, by the Mines and Quarries (Canteens) Order. A team of inspectors of the Ministry of Labour and National Service was empowered to ensure that a canteen was provided where required by an Order, and that it was "satisfactory" in terms of construction, size, equipment, and meals supplied. An advisory service was provided by the Ministry in the form of the Factory Canteen Advisors. These advisors, mostly women, who were selected for academic qualifications in nutrition or domestic science (home economics), or practical experience in managing commercial rest-aurants, hotels, or institutional canteens, were a source of help as well as control. They visited canteens, gave advice and assistance, and noted problems both to the employers and the Ministry's District Inspectors. Neither their (unannounced) visits, nor those of the Inspectors, resulted in any prosecutions. Nevertheless, a number of "Directions" were issued, over 100 in 1941, but they declined rapidly as the war progressed. A "Direction" was a formal order to comply with the legal provisions, persuasion having failed.(56)

Legislation, governmental encouragement and persuasion, and the conditions of a tight labor market with many workers far from home and working night shifts or other unusual hours, all helped to produce a rapid increase in the number of factory canteens, as shown in Table 1.

The rise and decline of bulding-site canteens reflects the pattern of wartime construction (military camps, hospitals, etc). Of more interest is the fact that factories employing fewer than 250 persons, and so not covered by the compulsory provisions of the Factories (Canteens) Order, established canteens at a more rapid rate than the larger factories. The reason for this difference is perhaps related to the pattern of usage of the canteens given in Table 2. This pattern, the reverse of that found in the United States, seems to reflect a strong preference for smaller more homelike canteens (restaurant eating was a habit little developed in Britain before World War II,

TABLE I

Growth in Number of Canteens
February 1941-March 1945

| Date | Factories | | Docks | Building Sites | Total |
	Employing Over 250	Employing Under 250			
Feb. 1941	1,650	—*	—	—	1,650
July 1941	2,580	1,439	70	460	4,549
Dec. 1941	3,165	2,530	110	787	6,592
Dec. 1942	4,340	4,141	160	868	9,509
Dec. 1943	4,877	5,704	176	782	11,535
Dec. 1944	5,046	6,584	179	245	12,054
Mar. 1945	5,069	6,772	177	227	12,245

* Data not available

Source: International Labour Office, Nutrition in Industry. Montreal: I.L.O., 1946, p. 142.

except among the affluent). It may also reflect the concentration of larger factories in the industrial north of England, where a long established tradition of bringing one's lunch to work prevailed. In such factories, too, class antagonisms were sharper, and canteens, whether run by the employer (as in 76 percent of cases) or by private caterers (21 percent), were suspect and liable to boycott. (The remaining 3 percent of canteens were run by workers' committees or joint committees.)(57)*

TABLE 2

Percentage of Employees Taking Hot Meals
March-September 1944

Number Employed	Day Shift	Night Shift
Over 1,000	28.9	35.8
500–1,000	26.8	47.5
250–500	39.8	50.2
Under 250	46.0	54.8

Source: International Labour Office, Nutrition in Industry. Montreal: I.L.O., 1946, p. 144

Elaborate and detailed measures were, then, taken by the state to ensure the availability of adequate inplant feeding facilities, and to supplement the industrial worker's rations in various other ways, such as through British Restaurants. The facilities were not always fully used, and not always available where they were needed. Taken together, however, those measures constituted a dramatic leap in the state's responsibility for the nutritional welfare of industrial workers. They were not relief measures aimed at the poor, or, in general, emergency measures for victims of enemy attack, but were aimed at the whole industrial work force as a regular, continuing means of helping to meet its nutritional needs. They were, in this sense, institutional and universal in conception, rather than residual and selective.

---

*The government, through the Chief Inspector of Factories, encouraged employers to take special steps to ensure that juvenile workers made full use of the canteens. Many firms responded, charging their young workers less than adults, or using a sliding scale based on age or pay, or contacting mothers to enlist their support. From 1943, the Ministry of Food made available a new product, National Milk-Cocoa, a mixture of dried milk, sugar, and cocoa devised by Drummond. It was to be sold to young mothers at not more than one penny for a third of a pint, but many firms supplied it free of charge.

Welfare Food Schemes: The Shift to Universalism

Those food programs for "vulnerable" sections of the population that have a clear continuity with the relief efforts of the 1930s did not disappear with the decline of poverty, unemployment, and food surpluses. On the contrary, they grew substantially and in doing so changed their character. The elements of Poor Law tradition, the emphasis on providing help only to those who could satisfy the state that they needed it, the opposition to taking over responsibilities and prerogatives from self-supporting families (and from local authorities and private corporations), in short, all the elements of economic and ideological conservatism that stood in the way of a universalist "welfare state" declined sharply. The danger to those "vulnerable" groups with special nutritional needs or risks — pregnant and lactating mothers, infants, and children — was seen as a danger facing all members of those groups and as arising not from individual weakness (or even economic forces affecting a minority), but from an external enemy threatening all. In taking on responsibility for the nutritional status of the whole population, as the state had done willy-nilly by undertaking to control the entire food supply, policymakers could hardly retain the welfare food programs for special groups on the old selective, residual basis. The need to maintain social solidarity and cohesiveness required the dropping of much of the invidious discrimination, between deserving and undeserving, self-supporting and dependent, givers and receivers, which characterized these programs in the 1930s.

To take the case of school meals: These had been provided, before July 1940, only to the "necessitous" and in practice only to a small proportion of those. Both the quality of the meals and the manner of their serving owed much to the deterrent principle enshrined in the Poor Law of 1834. As one local medical officer wrote in the mid thirties,

> Free dinners (lunches) unfortunately are still looked upon as a last resort; and many ill-nourished children of very necessitous parents, as well as children from less necessitous families, either do not wish to go to the dinners or the parents have an objection to their children receiving extra nourishment, although other forms of free medical treatment are accepted without any hesitation or feeling of degradation.(58)

Between 1935 and 1939 efforts were made to upgrade and expand the school meals service in response both to advances in nutritional knowledge and evidence of malnutrition in industrial areas. These efforts, in part a response to pressure from reformers like Eleanor Rathbone and LeGros Clark, increased the number of school lunches served daily in England and Wales from 143,000 in 1935 to nearly 160,000 in 1939. By July 1940 the disruptions of war had lowered the figure to 130,000.(59) In that month the Board of Education, with Treasury backing, decided to improve the quality of school meals and to provide them, as well as milk, for more children. Within a year the number of meals provided had doubled and the amount of school milk rose by 50 percent, more than recovering the ground lost during the first year of war.(60) In September 1941 the War Cabinet endorsed a plan to expand provision of school meals and milk still further by greatly increasing the national government's grants-in-aid to the local authorities.

The results were dramatic. By February 1945, 1,650,000 school lunches were provided daily in England and Wales, a tenfold increase over the July 1940 figure. One child in three now received the meals, compared with one in thirty in 1940. Fourteen percent of the children paid nothing for the lunches; the rest paid four or five pence per meal. While the policy aim of the War Cabinet to provide milk for every child at school was not achieved by the end of the war, there was an increase between July 1940 and February 1945 from 50 percent to 73 percent in the proportion of primary (elementary) and secondary school children receiving milk in school. The increase in the amount of milk drunk was still greater since many children were taking two thirds of a pint (imperial measure) per day, rather than one third.(61)

Severe wartime food shortages did not prevent improvement in the delivery of school meals and in their quality. The Ministry of Food granted exceptionally liberal allowances for school meals, especially of meat, liquid and dried milk, fats, preserves, and sugar. The Board, later Ministry, of Education provided the local authorities with the services of specialist inspectors, who advised them on standards and on planning and development of the program. The Ministry of Works built and equipped standard kitchens and dining facilities for the local authorities, although supplies of labor and materials were held up for a time by the needs of the American forces stationed in Britain.(62)

The school meals and milk programs thus shifted in the course of the war from being relief measures for the destitute to services for as many children as possible. From being highly selective programs for the very poor, they entered the universalist mainstream of the "welfare state." The milk-in-schools scheme extended even beyond the state sector in education to the private schools of the affluent and well-born. An element of selectivity was retained, however, in the free provision for those with very low incomes as opposed to the less-than-cost charges imposed on others.

School children were one of the priority classes to whom the government paid special attention. Another object of special concern was the population of expectant and nursing mothers and infants. As with school children (and, after 1943, adolescents working in factories), policy "went beyond maintaining the prewar diet and aimed at providing an optimum diet, regardless of purchasing power, for these special classes."(63)

The existence of the need for more milk, to reach mothers and children, and the awareness of that need enhanced by the propagandizing efforts of Sir John Boyd Orr and others, had not themselves produced serious action to meet the need. One month before the outbreak of the war, in August 1939, the Ministry of Health introduced a scheme to enable, but not compel, local authorities to provide cheap milk to mothers. The scheme was a failure. It involved a complicated and stigmatizing means test to determine whether mothers should receive milk free or at any price up to two pence (£.008). Local milk distributors opposed the scheme, and in some areas refused to cooperate, and local authorities disliked it because of its complexity and expense for them. The evacuation of major cities at the outbreak of the war made matters worse, as it moved potential beneficiaries out of the more "enlightened" local authorities' areas into those of the more "backward." In these early months of the war, the Ministry of Health lacked the authority and revenues to impose a uniform national program of subsidized milk consumption. Indeed, the national executive seemed unwilling and even unable to assert control in this area over local and sectional interests.

Five days after the evacuation of the British Expeditionary Force from Dunkirk, however, the Food Policy Committee of the War Cabinet gave the Ministers of Food and Health authority to work out a program for supplying cheap or free milk to mothers and children, without further reference to the Cabinet. The scheme was introduced in July. As Hammond says, "A social reform of the first magnitude, that at one time looked like languishing for months, if not years, was put into effect almost within days."(64)

The national milk scheme provided that every child under five years and all expectant and nursing mothers could receive one (imperial) pint of milk daily for two pence instead of the usual price of four-and-a-half pence. Infants under one year received the equivalent amount of milk in dried form. If the family income was below two pounds per week (plus six shillings a week for each nonearning dependent) the milk was free. The program was administered, unlike the 1939 scheme, by the Ministry of Food and its local food offices, and was financed wholly by the central government.(65)

The scheme was far more successful than officials at the Ministries of Food and Health had expected. They had underestimated the importance of purchasing power as an obstacle to milk consumption and exaggerated the unwillingness of the nonpoor to participate in a "welfare" program. By September 1940, 70 percent of the three-and-a-half million eligible mothers and children were participating. By September 1944, 19 out of 20 were taking part in the scheme. Both inflation and rising real incomes produced a remarkable fall in the proportion of recipients who did not pay anything for their milk. The drop, from nearly 30 percent in September 1940 to 2 percent in 1945, has been taken as one indicator of the "economic effects of the war in diminishing the amount of poverty among families containing expectant or nursing mothers and young children."(66)

Mothers and children who were covered by the national milk scheme also benefited from the provision of cheap or free orange juice and cod liver oil (or vitamin A and D tablets for those who could not take cod liver oil). This vitamin welfare scheme was introduced in December 1941, at first for children under two years, using blackcurrant syrup or purée as the vitamin C source. Orange juice, supplied under Lend-Lease, was substituted and coverage extended a few months later. The take-up rate for orange juice was low, however, and that for vitamin tablets and cod liver oil even lower. But the government's vigorous promotion of vitamins appears to have boosted the sale of commercial equivalents, thought by many to be superior, socially if not nutritionally.(67)

In terms of the state's taking responsibility for the nutritional adequacy of the nation's diet, these welfare food programs are of less significance than the nutritional aspects of general food policy, for the population as a whole or industrial workers in particular. Nevertheless, they clearly show the shift in social welfare practice and ideology, from the poor relief of the 1930s to the "welfare state" of the postwar years.

Nutrition and Inflation: Conflicting Priorities

Nutrition, we saw, was not at first a serious consideration in the government's food policy. In addition to the military question of the country's ability to withstand a blockade, that policy was above all concerned with inflation, and the related problem of industrial unrest. The appointment of the first Food Controller in World War I was, as F.H. Coller put it, a "reluctant sacrifice" on the "altar" of working class militancy.(68)

Pressure from below, resulting from a situation of acute labor shortage and the centrality of industrial production to the war effort, was felt as wage pressure. Food shortages raised prices and threatened to set off increased wage demands, pushing up costs in an inflationary spiral common to wartime. Failure to meet the demands could threaten, not only war production, but the political stability of the state.

Central control of wages and prices had been proposed by government planners as a wartime necessity since 1929, but the idea had steadily lost ground in face of feared trade union opposition. By 1939 official thinking, especially at the Ministry of Labour (but with some dissent in other departments), was along the lines summarized by H.M.D. Parker:

> If prices were held in check, representatives of employers and workers could be trusted, through the joint negotiating machinery which had brought the two sides closer together, to observe a realistic restraint in dealing with demands for higher wages; whereas any attempt to impose external control would lead to industrial unrest, which would both weaken morale and disrupt the whole economy of the country.(69)

While it had been thought that "profiteering" would be the main cause of food price rises, and that this could be checked with controls, by December 1939 that view was no longer tenable. The rise in import prices had gone so far that the Ministry of Food ("as much for want of time to revise its price schedules as anything else," according to Hammond) was losing a million pounds a week on its trading account.(70) To rectify this situation would have required an immediate rise of 12 points in the official cost of living index and that, it was feared, would wreck the government's strategy of getting official union backing for a policy of wage restraint. Thus even a reluctant Treasury was driven in the direction of (supposedly "temporary") food subsidies and price stabilization.(71)

The evolution and details of the bargain struck with labor (price stabilization in return for wage restraint) need not concern us here, but it is worth noting how the cost-of-living index became a device for deflecting working-class pressure, in short, for cheating labor out of its part of the deal. The working-class cost-of-living index was central to the bargain because in many industries wages were fixed with reference to it, while in others it formed the basis of collective bargaining.

Henry Smith, in his 1937 analysis of Retail Distribution, observed of the index that it was "devoted to the somewhat peculiar purpose of ascertaining what the value of money would be to a hypothetical and extremely conservative working-class family and the habits of consumption to which it was accustomed in 1914."(72) Some items of working-class consumption, such as beer, wines, spirits, and electricity were omitted altogether from the index. Others, such as tobacco, were heavily underweighted in relation to actual consumption in 1939. Eggs, on the other hand, were an altogether disproportionate part of the index in light of the limited quantities available in wartime.

Using these peculiarities to its advantage, the government was able to manipulate retail prices so as to keep down the official cost of living for the working class, as reflected in the index. Eggs, for example, were heavily subsidized, while beer and tobacco were heavily taxed. Far from being an additional "burden" on the

Treasury, the ever-increasing cost of food subsidies was borne out of indirect and highly regressive taxation. This "pious fraud," as Hammond calls it, enabled the state to hold down wages and save its price stabilization policy in face of a very tight labor market.(73) Had the index reflected working-class consumption patterns in war-time in the 1940s, and had the government been less willing to take advantage of its imperfections as a statistical instrument, it is highly unlikely that the policy of controlling inflation at the expense of working-class living standards could have survived.

While good nutritional reasons could be advanced (and by some welfare-minded officials were advanced) for taxing tobacco and subsidizing eggs, the government's creative use of bad statistics was motivated not by a desire to aid the family or maintain health standards, but simply by the aim of controlling inflation. The net effect of these tax and food subsidy policies, in terms of nutrition, inflation, or real living standards, is uncertain. Hammond observes,

> There were, of course, people who, through poverty or inclination, paid less in taxes than the average cost per head of the general food subsidies and thus could be said to benefit from them — nonsmokers with large families and old-age pensioners, for example. But this does not alter the general principle that, so far from being a measure designed to promote welfare, the subsidies were a sacrifice of the welfare principle to one deemed more important, namely, the prevention of inflation.(74)

Eggs (and many other basic foodstuffs) were, in any case, in short supply and rigidly controlled. Tobacco and alcohol, on the other hand, were unrationed. One clear result of government policy, then, was that consumption of the latter commodities increased to the point where it absorbed a large part of the additional real earnings that workers derived from their longer hours of work. The economic historian Alan Milward, discussing the difficulties of the concept of a real wage in so administered an economy, asks what could be bought for the increased real wage. "In Britain," he argues, "the answer was tobacco and alcohol."(75)

CONCLUSION

Critics of the first edition of <u>Food, Health, and Income</u> said that it was utopian to adopt a dietary standard that would make possible good health as opposed to mere survival. Boyd Orr responded in the second edition (1937) as follows:

> In animal husbandry, an optimum standard, far from being utopian, is regarded as good practice. Every intelligent stock

farmer in rearing animals tries to get a minimum diet for maximum health and physical fitness. A suggestion that he should use a lower standard would be regarded as absurd. If children of the three lower groups were reared for profit like young farm stock, giving them a diet below the requirements for health would be financially unsound. Unfortunately, the health and physical fitness of the rising generation are not marketable commodities which can be assessed in terms of money.

From the point of view of the State, the adoption of a standard of diet lower than the optimum is uneconomic. It leads to a great amount of preventable disease and ill-health which lay a heavy burden on the State, and on the public-spirited citizens who support hospitals and other charitable organizations. . . .A few years hence when the connection between the poor feeding of mothers and children and subsequent poor physique and ill-health is as clearly recognized as the connection between a contaminated water supply and cholera, the suggestion that a diet fully adequate to health should be available for everyone will be regarded as reasonable and in accordance with common sense, as is the preservation of our domestic water supply from pollution.(76)

There was indeed a growing recognition of the connection between nutrition and health in the 1930s, and of the social costs of malnutrition and disease. But labor-power is in fact a "marketable commodity," and when war produced a scarcity of it, the state became much more heavily involved in measures to conserve the health and physical fitness of present and future workers. The growth of state action in this area was not simply a matter of economic calculation, however. Military success, rather than profits, was the immediate overriding priority, and it depended upon the morale and loyalty as well as the physical fitness of the nation's manpower. Both kinds of consideration found expression in the extensiveness and universalism of the state's response to the problems of food and nutrition in a total war.

The overall impact of that response is difficult to assess, but one indication is that the percentage of personal disposable income spent on food fell during the war from 29 percent to 23.4 percent, whereas in the more prosperous United States, where food retail prices were not subsidized and rationing was less strict or comprehensive, food costs as a proportion of total expenditure increased from 24.3 percent in 1940 to 30.6 percent in 1943.(77) As Boyd Orr and David Lubbock observed in 1940, "The difficulty in war is the same as it was in peacetime, not one of supply but one of more equal distribution of the food which is available."(78) An effect of government policy was to redistribute a smaller national food supply so that the average level of health and nutrition was improved.(79)

War had in this sense stimulated a more efficient allocation of scarce resources, mediated by the state.

Capitalist resistances to state intervention, which was strong while labor was weak and labor power plentiful in the 1930s, gave way under pressure of war. There was, as Boyd Orr recognized in 1937, a collective interest, embodied in the state, in the adequate nutrition of the populace. It took the crisis of total war to enforce this recognition on the representatives of capital.

Contemporaries like Titmuss and Hammond saw the growth of the state's responsibility for the nation's food and nutrition as a revolutionary change. At the end of the 1940s, when Titmuss wrote Problems of Social Policy, it appeared that the social solidarity and collective responsibility imposed by war had brought about a permanent shift in the relations of private capital and the state. State controls and rationing were being phased out, but a range of universal provisions remained, including school meals and milk, subsidized milk and orange juice for mothers and young children, and subsidized food prices for all. These developments seemed part of a larger network of services and provisions, which together provided a measure of economic security and social dignity to all. It came to be known as the "welfare state" and seemed to represent a fundamental subordination of market forces to social control, a final rejection of the harshness and greed of laissez faire and Poor Law. It seemed irreversible, like the defeat of feudalism.

Much of Titmuss's later work constitutes a kind of rearguard action, a defense of the achievements of the welfare state of the 1940s and a plea for their extension even in the face of the social, economic, and ideological forces he saw as threatening them. The optimism that pervades Problems of Social Policy is absent from his later writing. "We exaggerated the trend toward equality during the Second World War in respect to income, employment and other factors," he reflected in 1966, "...and optimistically projected short-term trends into the future."(80)

The social policy developments of the 1940s seemed less revolutionary and less adequate in the perspective of later years. They also seemed less permanent, as social provisions, including food and nutrition programs, were cut back, made increasingly selective, or eliminated.(81) Nevertheless, the crisis of war had brought about an expansion of the state's role in the economy and society. There was to be no return to prewar levels of state intervention and control. The postwar welfare state was no less capitalist, but it was, and has remained, more corporatist.(82) The state played a more positive role in enforcing general capitalist interests on individual capitals during the war, by comparison both with the 1930s and with the American state during World War II. It continued in the postwar period to organize both the social conditions for capital accumulation and the accumulation process itself, not to the same degree as during the war, but to a greater extent than ever before it.

NOTES

(1) For contrasting views, see E.J. Hobsbawm, "British Standard of Living," and R.M. Hartwell, "Rising Standard of Living."

(2) John Boyd Orr, Food and the People, p. 15.

(3) Richard M. Titmuss, Problems of Social Policy, p. 514, n. 2.

(4) Sir Arthur S. MacNalty, ed., The Civilian Health and Medical Services, vol. I, p. 152.

(5) Titmuss, Problems, p. 511; Sir William Crawford and H. Broadley, The People's Food, p. 209; John Burnett, Plenty and Want, p. 254.

(6) Angus Calder, The People's War, p. 132.

(7) R.J. Hammond, Food and Agriculture, p. 141; John Boyd Orr, Food, Health and Income; UK Ministry of Health, Advisory Committee on Nutrition: First Report.

(8) Orr, Food, Health and Income, p. 18; Burnett, Plenty and Want, p. 237; John Stevenson, Social Conditions in Britain, p. 127.

(9) Orr, Food, Health and Income, p. 44.

(10) Ibid, pp. 44-49, 55-56

(11) G.C.M. M'Gonigle and J. Kirby, Poverty and Public Health.

(12) Derek Fraser, The Evolution of the British Welfare State, p. 180.

(13) Drummond and Wilbraham, Englishman's Food, p. 444.

(14) Orr, Food, Health and Income, p. 7.

(15) British Medical Association, Inquiry into Minimum Weekly Expenditure.

(16) John Boyd Orr and D. Lubbock, Feeding the People in Wartime.

(17) Crawford and Broadley, People's Food, pp. 122-61.

(18) Burnett, Plenty and Want, pp. 233-34.

(19) "An Attack on Maternal Mortality," Lancet, July 6, 1935, p. 50.

(20) Burnett, Plenty and Want, p. 241.

(21) Pilgrim Trust, Men Without Work.

(22) Drummond and Wilbraham, Englishman's Food, p. 448; Burnett, Plenty and Want, p. 256.

(23) Titmuss, Problems, p. 507; Burnett, Plenty and Want, p. 256.

(24) The pressure for a "marriage of health and agriculture," discussed in the following chapter, came mainly from the primary food-producing countries, notably Australia and the United States.

(25) Eric Roll, Combined Food Board, p. 8.

(26) Hammond, Food and Agriculture, p. 12.

(27) Ibid., pp. 9-10; idem, Food, vol. I, pp. 10-11; William Beveridge, Power and Influence, pp. 240-44.

(28) Hammond, Food and Agriculture, p. 140.

(29) Ibid, p. 140.

(30) Idem, Food, vol. I, p. 218.

(31) Burnett, Plenty and Want, p. 259.

(32) Drummond and Wilbraham, Englishman's Food, pp. 449-53.

(33) Hammond, Food and Agriculture, p. 143.

(34) Ibid, pp. 243-44.

(35) Lord Woolton, Memoirs, p. 1.

(36) Hammond, Food, vol. I, p. 218.

(37) UK Ministry of Health, On the State of Public Health, pp. 14-21, 58-59.

(38) Roll, Combined Food Board, p. 8.

(39) Calder, People's War, p. 132.

(40) Ibid, p. 318; UK Ministry of Food, How Britain Was Fed in Wartime.

(41) Alan S. Milward, War, Economy and Society, p. 233.

(42) Calder, People's War, p. 440; see also UK Ministry of Food, How Britain Was Fed, pp. 25-41.

(43) Drummond and Wilbraham, Englishman's Food, p. 454.

(44) The Times (London), June 20, 1939. Cited by Titmuss, Problems, p. 516.

(45) UK Ministry of Health, On the State of Public Health, pp. 14-21, 58-59; Titmuss, Problems, pp. 517-19.

(46) See J.R. Marrack, "Investigations of Human Nutrition"; British Medical Association, Report of the Committee on Nutrition, London, 1950.

(47) Hammond, Food and Agriculture, p. 157.

(48) On the state of morale see especially Calder, People's War, pp. 126, 247-58, passim; Tom Harrison, Living Through the Blitz; William Rankin, "What Dunkirk Spirit?" Useful contemporary accounts include Ritchie Calder, Lesson of London; Negley Farson, Bomber's Moon; Harold Nicolson, Diaries and Letters.

(49) Quoted by Hammond, Food and Agriculture, p. 173.

(50) Hammond, Food and Agriculture, p. 173, 175.

(51) Parliamentary Debates, House of Commons, May 7, 1941, vol. 371, col. 850.

(52) Calder, People's War, p. 446.

(53) William Foster, John Company, p. 142.

(54) Annual Report of H.M. Chief Inspector of Factories for 1918, p. 31.

(55) Calder, People's War, p. 446. The Ministry of Labour guessed the number of industrial canteens on outbreak of war to have been about 2,000. UK Ministry of Labour and National Service, First Annual Report, 1943-1944, p. 14.

(56) International Labour Office (ILO), Nutrition in Industry, p. 143; see also ibid., pp. 135-42.

(57) ILO, Nutrition in Industry, p. 154; Mass Observation, People in Production, pp. 274-75.

(58) Quoted by F. LeGros Clark, Social History of School Meals Service, p. 14. See also Titmuss, Problems p. 509.

(59)   Titmuss, Problems, p. 510.

(60)   Ibid.

(61)   Ibid.

(62)   Ministry of Health, On the State of Public Health, p. 117; Clark, School Meals Service, p. 23.

(63)   UK Ministry of Health, On the State of Public Health, p. 117.

(64)   Hammond, Food, vol. I, pp. 101-2.

(65)   Titmuss, Problems, p. 511.

(66)   Titmuss, Problems, p. 512; Calder, People's War, p. 444.

(67)   Hammond, Food and Agriculture, p. 149.

(68)   F.H. Coller, State Trading Adventure, p. 149.

(69)   Parker, Manpower, p. 424.

(70)   Hammond, Food and Agriculture, p. 152.

(71)   Ibid.

(72)   Henry Smith, Retail Distribution, p. 85.

(73)   Hammond, Food and Agriculture, p. 153.

(74)   Ibid., p. 154.

(75)   Milward, War, Economy and Society, p. 239.

(76)   Orr, Food, Health and Income, pp. 7-8.

(77)   Milward, War, Economy and Society, p. 286. Cf. E.F. Nash, "Wartime Control of Food and Agricultural Prices," p. 201; J.D. Black and C.A. Gibbons, "The War and American Agriculture."

(78)   Orr and Lubbock, Feeding the People in Wartime, p. 69.

(79)   Hammond, Food, vol. I, pp. 368-71; Mancur Olson, Jr., Economics of Wartime Shortage, p. 29.

(80)   Titmuss, Commitment to Welfare, p. 163.

(81)   Ibid, pp. 153-65; Marwick, Britain in the Century of Total War, pp.   389-92, 430-47; Jim Kincaid, "Decline of the Welfare State."

(82)   See, for example, Nigel Harris, Competition and the Corporate Society; Michael Kidron, Western Capitalism Since the War; Leo Panitch, Social Democracy and Industrial Militancy; Andrew Shonfield, Modern Capitalism; Harold Wilensky, The "New Corporatism," Centralization, and the Welfare State.

5

WAR AND NUTRITION: THE UNITED STATES

The American government played a more active role than the British with regard to nutrition in the 1930s. It not only sponsored much research and education, but also adapted its relief policy so as to improve the nutritional status of the destitute while helping farmers dispose of their surplus production. As in Britain, World War II changed the definition of the problem, from relief of the destitute and starving, combined with absorption of the agricultural surplus, to one of ensuring the health and efficiency of the population as a whole. Attempts to deal with the problem, however, revealed the weakness and disunity within the American state, its inability to establish anything equal to the prevailing British level of autonomy and authority with regard to specific interests. Although subject to many of the same pressures and tendencies, the United States was less vulnerable in terms of the nutritional status of its population and in other respects. It could afford a lower level of state autonomization. Food shortages were much less severe than in Britain, but they had a very different impact on welfare food programs, a difference suggestive of weaker pressures for universalism in social welfare.

THE 1930s: NUTRITION AND RELIEF

In the United States, as in Britain, the Depression, with its mass unemployment and hunger, stimulated concern about nutrition. Whereas the translation of such concern into state action was inhibited in Britain by a political and economic conservatism that sought to limit government spending, in the United States, it was affected by other forces.

The Depression hit the United States harder than Britain, and it produced a higher degree of state autonomization in response. The relative strength and autonomy of the national executive increased dramatically under Roosevelt, who was able in his first administration to push through his far-reaching New Deal legislation with remarkably little opposition. As in Germany, though with very different results for the working class, capitalists had been forced to give the state its head under a strong national leader, in the hope that it would preserve and restore the conditions in which capital could be accumulated. Roosevelt, like Hitler, was pragmatic in his approach to economic matters, and was not hamstrung by the prevailing fiscal orthodoxy.(1)

Not only was the general political and economic situation in the United States different from that in Britain, but the position and importance of agriculture in the two countries were also in sharp contrast. Whereas Britain, as an agricultural importer, benefitted from the world slump in food prices, the United States was faced with the political embarrassment of large food surpluses amidst hunger and malnutrition. Food was going to waste or being destroyed while thousands went hungry. The American government, therefore, did not share the complacency of the British with regard to food prices or malnutrition. On the contrary, it sought a "marriage" between nutrition and agriculture both domestically and, together with another primary food producer, Australia, internationally, through the League of Nations. Most of the important nutritional research, whether into human requirements for nutrition, or dietary surveys, was sponsored by the government, which also became increasingly concerned with nutritional education. In its search for constructive and politically acceptable ways of disposing of the agricultural surplus without depressing farmers' prices, the U.S. Department of Agriculture also became heavily involved in relief policy.

Agriculture was, then, much more important, politically and economically, for the United States than for Britain, and its plight in the 1930s provided a stimulus for state involvement in the problem of malnutrition. Rather, the stimulus derived from the problem of political illegitimacy resulting from the measures taken to deal with that plight. The demands of economic efficiency (the accumulation or efficiency function of the state) pulled policy in the direction of disposing of the agricultural surplus in ways which would not disrupt the market. But state involvement in destroying or limiting food supplies in a situation of mass hunger posed obvious problems of legitimation. While millions went hungry or poorly nourished, the Agricultural Adjustment Administration vigorously pursued a policy of trying to restrict farm output. Pigs were being slaughtered in order to maintain prices at levels which the unemployed could not afford.(2) In face of the outcry elicited by those policies, the government decided to buy up some of the surplus for distribution to the poor. Economic and political needs, efficiency, and legitimation could thus be served at the same time. Agriculture and relief officials together, in symbolic unity, led by Henry Wallace, Secretary of Agriculture, and Harry Hopkins, administrator of the Federal Emergency Relief Administration (FERA), incorporated the Federal Surplus Relief Corporation in October 1933.(3) The corporation, which purchased surplus commodities and distributed them to state and local relief agencies, was under the direction of the FERA administrator, Hopkins. In 1936, however, its name was changed to Federal Surplus Commodities Corporation and it was placed under the direction of the Department of Agriculture and the presidency of Chester Davis, administrator of the Agricultural Adjustment Administration(4).

This change of names and control not only signified Roosevelt's desire to get the federal government out of the business of temporary relief; the shift also represented the primary importance attached to surplus disposal, that is, to agricultural interests. For if a marriage between nutrition and agriculture indeed took place in the 1930s, it was a very unequal relationship, a marriage of convenience in which the interests of agriculture clearly took precedence. As agriculture stimulated governmental interest in nutrition, it also shaped and limited it.

RESEARCH AND EDUCATION

By the 1930s, knowledge about nutritional needs was becoming widespread. Research carried out in the first three decades of the century had led to the discovery of vitamins (and a growing knowledge of their nature and identities), of the amino acids, and of certain minerals. The "newer knowledge of nutrition" – as the leading nutritional scientist Elmer V. McCollum called it in his book of that title – pointed, among other things, to the need for an adequate supply of "protective foods."(5) This term, coined by McCollum in 1918 and given very wide currency in the 1930s, referred to foods rich in calcium and vitamins A and C, such as milk and certain fruits and vegetables. The importance of vitamin D and certain elements of the B complex, as well as the loss of these and other nutrients in the processing of staples like white flour, was increasingly understood.

Armed with this knowledge, researchers were well equipped to establish the nature and extent of malnutrition in the United States. Early studies, such as those of mining areas carried out by the U.S. Children's Bureau in the early 1930s, showed that relief efforts at that time were not preventing severe undernourishment, and even starvation.(6) A New York City study in 1935 showed that even there, with the highest per capita relief expenditure of any large city, the food allowance was insufficient to maintain health in 30 of the 34 precincts.(7) Official reports and journalistic exposés of hunger, such as Paul DeKruif's Why Keep Them Alive? and Maxine Davis's Atlantic Monthly article, "Hungry Children," reinforced the pressure for more systematic studies.

In 1933, Hazel K. Stiebeling, senior food economist at the Bureau of Home Economics (USDA), and Medora Ward produced a bulletin, Diets at Four Levels of Nutritive Content and Cost, which received wide attention. Based on the nutritional standards developed in the 1920s by Henry C. Sherman and other scientists, they presented four model diets, the most meager of them being a restricted diet for emergency use, costing at 1931-1932 prices $61 per year, for one person. The pamphlet was intended for use by welfare workers, teachers, and others as an educational tool. It was popularized by Gove Hambidge in Your Meals and Your Money, in 1934. It also formed the basis for later studies, which established a working pattern of amounts of nutrients and food required daily for individuals of different ages, sex, and activity levels. In 1936, an attempt was made to determine the extent of malnutrition in the United States. The Bureau of Home Economics and Bureau of Labor Statistics, in collaboration with the National Resources Committee, the Central Statistical Board, and the WPA, carried out a nation-wide study of consumer purchases and their nutritional adequacy, directed by Stiebeling. Their negative findings reinforced official concern and, in the context of the United States' impending entry into a world war, prompted Roosevelt to call the National Nutrition Conference for Defense in May 1941.(8)

Two broad conclusions could be drawn from the great volume of research sponsored in the 1930s by the Department of Agriculture, Public Health Service, Children's Bureau, and other government agencies. One was that a third to a half of the nation was subsisting on diets that were seriously inadequate according to existing standards.(9) The other was that "an adequate or superior diet for all the nation's population would require more rather than fewer acres in production, though the pattern of production would be somewhat different."(10) These findings, and the growing feeling that more attention needed to be given to supplying adequate food for all, instead of curtailing production, had some influence, according to Murray R. Benedict, "among the more forward-looking members of the official Washington staff in agriculture."(11) A fundamental shift in policy was not forthcoming, however, and, as Benedict says, "Farm groups and most agricultural officials still thought in terms of surpluses of production rather than deficits in consumption."(12)

To a much greater extent than in Britain, though still on a modest scale, attempts were made to educate people in the "newer knowledge of nutrition," and to utilize nutritionists in program planning. The Department of Agriculture, through the home demon-stration agents of the Extension Service, had been carrying on educational work among the rural poor since the 1920s, providing instruction not only in human nutrition, but also in techniques of food raising.(13) This work was expanded in the 1930s to provide additional instruction to increased numbers of poor and dependent families. Gladys Baker describes how home demonstration agents and state extension specialists in South Carolina trained assistants — financed by WPA funds — to carry on "special nutrition work with needy families."(14) In North Carolina, relief funds were used for emergency home demonstration agents.(15) Many states and some cities began to hire nutritionists in small numbers.(16)

Educational efforts were directed mainly at the poor because their malnutrition was widely believed to result from their ignorance. If they used their money more wisely, it was argued, they would be able to eat adequately and avoid any nutritional deficiency. While some writers and groups, especially those representing labor organizations or liberal politics, saw low purchasing power as the root cause of malnutrition, and many, including social workers, blamed both ignorance and poverty, the dominant view was that expressed by leaders of the AMA like James McLester and Morris Fishbein.(17) That view was that no amount of increased purchasing power would help unless people learned to select their food purchases wisely. "People must also learn," Fishbein added, "to spend money on food rather than on some other matters that appeal to the American pocketbook," like cigarettes, gasoline, clothing, soft drinks, or improved housing.(18)

While the state thus became quite heavily involved in nutritional education as well as research, its officers sometimes had to tread carefully in face of suspicion and hostility from food processors. When meatpackers protested in 1931 against a radio broadcast of the U.S. Public Health Service, which advised people to eat less meat in hot weather, the service was ordered to submit all future broadcasts to the Secretary of the Treasury for censorship. The millers campaigned to have unfair references to white bread expunged from school textbooks and, objecting to the publication, Diets at Four Levels of Nutritive Content and Cost, had a rider attached to a 1934 agricultural appropriation bill stating that no one receiving funds from USDA should be allowed to make derogatory statements about any "wholesome" food. This provision was dropped in the face of strong protests by those concerned with nutritional education.(19)

NUTRITION AND RELIEF POLICY

The Great Depression, with its mass unemployment and drought, challenged several long-standing beliefs and attitudes about poor relief. Social workers and their sponsors had traditionally favored provision of relief in kind rather than in cash. The underlying assumption was that clients could not be trusted to spend their money wisely, and that a degree of social control over their behavior was both in their own interests and implicit in their dependency. Josephine C. Brown, in her study of Public Relief 1929-1939, describes the emergence of a "democratic" philosophy in unemployment relief, resulting from a change of social work clientele during and following World War I (the Home Service of the American Red Cross, which provided social work services not to the dependent poor but to servicemen and their families) and the influence of psychiatry.

This "new democratic approach to people,"(20) taught in progressive social work schools and agencies in the 1920s, was reinforced by the swelling of the relief rolls, from the fall of 1929, with new millions of the unemployed. "Here the average relief applicant was so obviously competent and accustomed to managing his own affairs and supporting himself in a normal way that it was utterly useless and absurd to pretend that he was at fault, and a self-made pauper."(21)

Relief in kind persisted in many areas, in part because of disorganization and absence of alternatives, in part because of the persistence of traditional attitudes to the dependent poor. In the early 1930s especially, food was often the only form of relief available, and it was dispensed in a variety of ways, including the commissary (a relief store in which packages of food and sometimes clothing were given away), soup kitchens, and other "primitive" methods. Nevertheless, the official policy of the federal government, under the leadership of Harry Hopkins, was to press for work relief rather than direct relief, and for relief in cash rather than in kind. In March 1934, the order was issued that all work relief was to be paid in cash, but direct relief continued to be paid in kind or cash according to the policies of the state and local relief administrations. The FERA strongly recommended cash payments, both as preserving the normal responsibility of the family for its own purchases, and because it maintained existing channels of retail trade instead of substituting for them.(22)

The question of what form relief should take was a difficult and controversial matter, in which the federal relief administration took a clear position and pressed for its acceptance at the state and local level. Into this situation entered the Federal Surplus Relief Corporation, and later the Federal Surplus Commodities Corporation, pursuing the opposite principle. The contradiction is well described by Brown, writing in 1940:

With the establishment of the new surplus commodities system in October of that year (1933) the Federal Administration, which was encouraging localities to give direct relief in cash and insisting, in the spring of 1934, that all work relief wages be paid by cash or check, continued to give relief in kind through a program which was financed almost entirely by Federal funds and was entirely under Federal control. This distribution of surplus commodities not only constituted relief in kind, but "package" or "basket" relief handed out through commissaries or at the corner grocery store where the recipients were bound to be publicly marked as "reliefers" to all their neighborhood. In order to regulate prices and take surplus goods off the market, the Federal Administration has been willing for six years to give direct Federal relief of the most demoralizing and stigmatizing type.(23)

This form of relief was to persist for over 30 years more. If the new "democratic principle" in unemployment relief was undermined by the surplus commodities program, perhaps the interests of nutrition were served. To some extent this appears to be the case, but not because the purchase and distribution of surplus foods was planned to ensure a balanced and nutritionally adequate diet. On the contrary, as Howard P. Davis, then a high official within the Surplus Marketing Administration (successor to the FSCC), wrote in 1959, "Because conditions in the farm market determine the kinds and volume of surplus food the Department acquires, the donation program cannot be geared in any important degree to the preferences or nutritional needs of the recipients."(24)

Nevertheless, the foods purchased for distribution in the late 1930s were both nutritious and, for the most part, positive additions to the standard high energy staple diet of the poor. They included prominently, grapefruit, prunes, eggs, oranges and various other fruits, vegetables, and dairy products.(25) Part of the nutritional value of the program was in changing food habits and expectations, leading, for instance, to a substantially increased use among low income groups of dry and whole milk. Grapefruit and other citrus fruits also became customary to many who had previously been unfamiliar with them. (Several versions were current of the story of the boiled grapefruit: the relief recipient or school meals manager tells of boiling grapefruit for hours and hours but still finding them tough.(26)) Insofar as surpluses did include staples like flour, rice, and beans, their donation freed recipient income that would have normally been spent on these foods, permitting the purchase of meat, vegetables, or dairy products. However, the same effect could have been achieved by the donation of cash. In any case, the federal surplus commodities program, while probably having some nutritional benefits for recipients, was clearly not shaped or designed for that purpose. The benefits were contingent on whatever surpluses happened to be available.

The same was true of the Food Stamp program, introduced by Milo Perkins, head of the FSCC, in May 1939, first in Rochester, New York, and later in other cities. Under this plan, for every one dollar orange stamp bought at face value by relief clients, a 50-cent blue stamp was given free. The orange stamps could be exchanged at participating stores for essentially any food, but the blue stamps had to be used for foods on the list of those designated by the Secretary of Agriculture as surplus. The list consisted, in May 1939, of flour, cornmeal, dried beans, butter, eggs, and citrus fruits, and changed from time to time subsequently.(27) The program was popular both with recipients, who were able to exercise a wider freedom of choice than if commodities were donated directly, and with retailers, whose services were being used instead of bypassed.(28) The primary purpose of the program, however, was to help shift the agricultural surplus and prevent the price-depressing effects of overproduction and the politically damaging effects of food destruction amidst hunger. As a stimulant to the agricultural economy, the program was probably not very effective, but that was nevertheless its main point.(29) In any case, the program arose out of, and derived its rationale from, the existence of an agricultural surplus, a point of some significance when the surplus disappeared.

The Agriculture Department's other main outlet for surplus food was the school lunch program. Prior to the 1930s, school lunches had developed more as a matter of convenience than of welfare, notwithstanding their welfare origins in the industrial schools of the Children's Aid Society. They were usually self-supporting and more common in high schools than at the primary level. A 1918 survey of 86 cities found some provision for lunches in high schools in 76 percent of the cities, as opposed to 25 percent for elementary schools.(30) The Department of Agriculture and state extension workers became involved in providing plans and dietary advice in the setting up of lunch plans in rural schools. The nutritional and educational possibilities of school lunches became increasingly attractive to school officials and others.

In the 1930s, the emphasis shifted to the feeding of hungry children. School lunches became, in many cases, a part of poor relief. The states became involved with funding for lunches for needy schoolchildren. In 1934, New York State appropriated $100,000 of relief funds for free lunches and milk for poor children.(31)

In 1932 and 1933, the federal government, in the form of the Reconstruction Finance Corporation, first aided school lunch programs by making loans to several Missouri towns to pay the labor costs of preparing and serving lunches. Under Roosevelt this type of assistance was extended by the Civil Works and Federal Emergency Relief Administrations. By the end of 1934, it had reached 39 states, and financed the employment of 7,400.(32) The National Youth Administration provided some labor for operating school lunch programs, fresh and processed vegetables from their gardening and canning projects, and tables, chairs, and other equipment that they had constructed. From 1935, a major federal contribution to the school lunch programs was made by the Works Progress Administra tion. Through the WPA, the federal government provided labor and trained supervision, established standards, and made federal inspection a requirement.(33)

Section 32 of Public Law 320, 74th Congress, passed in August 1935, provided a permanent annual appropriation, derived from customs receipts, to the Agriculture Department, for the general purpose of expanding markets for agricultural commodities. It was under this legislation that surplus foods were bought and distributed to, among other beneficiaries, nonprofit school lunch programs. In 1938, according to Marvin M. Sandstrom, the FSCC provided supplies for lunches to 9,100 schools serving about 540,000 students, and during 1939-1940 the program was further expanded, reaching 2.5 million children in 1940.(34) The food was allocated to schools on the basis of the number of children "certified" as needy or undernourished. Such children were to be fed free of charge.

Supplementing the school lunch program, a "penny milk program" begun in 1939 on a trial basis in 15 Chicago schools, was extended to New York City in October 1940; by the end of the 1941-1942 school year, it was operating in 99 areas and providing milk daily for 731,000 children.(35) Under this scheme, designed both to increase producer income and to raise the milk consumption of needy children, the Secretary of Agriculture subsidized milk producers so that they could sell milk to schools at one cent per half pint. The milk was then sold to the children at the same price, with teachers and others donating money to provide free milk for those without the requisite penny. (Some milk was also sold at a subsidized low price to families in need.)(36)

As it developed and expanded in the 1930s, the school lunch program exhibited some familiar themes. It had a relief orientation, and it was an outlet for the agricultural surplus. It also provided a form of work relief for its employees. Nutritional and educational goals were stressed by school administrators, who sought control of the programs, and local sponsoring groups, governmental or voluntary, supplemented the surplus foods to provide a balanced diet. However, war would knock away two of the program's props, the agricultural surplus and work relief, placing the program in jeopardy.

WORLD WAR II

Weakness of the State

Entry by the United States into World War II dictated a substantial shift in the state's policy toward nutrition and agriculture. Existing farm policy, together with the programs, agencies, and attitudes in which it found expression, was geared to protect the farmer against low prices. War, it was feared, would simply exacerbate the problems of the 1930s, a prognosis that the decline of farm prices in 1940 appeared to confirm.(37) The reversal of policy, in the direction of increasing production, took place more slowly in agriculture than in other areas. Benedict suggests some of the reasons for this early inertia:

> The ways of thinking and the kinds of laws developed in the 1930s were not easily put aside. The fear of surpluses was more evident than the fear of shortages. Congressmen continued to stress protection of the farmer against low prices, and the men in charge of the agricultural programs moved cautiously. The administrators who headed the nonagricultural war agencies were, generally speaking, brought in for the specific purpose of stepping up and changing production. Agriculture, on the other hand, already had a large bureaucracy consisting of men who for years had been fighting to keep production down and prices up. Many were career men who felt that if they erred too greatly on the side of excess production they themselves would later be the chief targets of farmer and public criticism.(38)

The needs of the new, wartime situation, in particular the control of inflation and prevention of serious food shortages, were thus superimposed on patterns of thinking and organization that had been developed to meet quite opposite needs. Nutrition had been a concern of the state in the context of the need to dispose of the agricultural surplus in ways that would not be economically or politically disruptive. Nutritional policy provided an element of legitimation for an agricultural policy of cutting back food production in a country where millions went hungry. (Conservation, however, had been the main legitimating argument for reducing agricultural production.)(39) Food shortages, full employment, and increased consumer purchasing power now threatened to break up the "marriage" of nutrition and agriculture. At the same time nutrition emerged into new prominence as a direct and immediate concern of the state, independent of any need to dispose of surplus food or prevent starvation of the destitute.

The need now was for a healthy military and work force capable of sustaining a total and perhaps prolonged war. Of the first million men examined under the Selective Service system instituted in 1940, Brigadier-General Lewis B. Hershey told the National Nutrition Conference, about 40 percent were rejected as unfit for military service, and about a third of these rejections were attributed to the effects of nutritional deficiencies.(40) Standards for the medical examination varied according to the manpower requirements of the armed services, which were at their highest before Pearl Harbor, but Hershey's figure was widely publicized and was a catalyst for official concern about nutrition. Draft rejection rates may not have been a reliable index of the national health,(41) but they strongly underlined the importance of the nutritional status of the population for the state's ability to conduct a major war.

That point was taken up by the Subcommittee on Health and Education of the Senate Committee on Education and Labor. Senator Claude Pepper, chairman of the subcommittee, said at hearings held in the war-industry town of Pascagoula, Mississippi:

> This committee, therefore, has as one of its objectives the discovery of the conditions which produced so high a number of rejections from the military service. No nation is stronger than its people. We have found that the greatest resource we have is our manpower, the ability of our people to fight and to work for their country. So we are interested in anything that has to do with the eligibility and fitness of the citizenship (sic) of this country to wage war and to maintain the production necessary for waging war.(42)

In addition to the hearings in Pascagoula, the subcommittee also heard a great deal of testimony in Washington, including that of senior officers in the armed services concerned with selective service, veterans' affairs, and army and navy medical services. They gave the subcommittee, in the words of Rilla Schroeder, Survey's Washington correspondent, "an appalling picture of the health and general physical condition of American youth."(43)

Official concern about nutrition also found expression in the establishment of many new committees at the federal, state, and local level, and in Roosevelt's calling the first presidential conference on nutrition. The issue was raised early by the National Defense Advisory Commission, created by President Roosevelt in 1940, which appointed an advisor on nutrition. Paul V. McNutt, Federal Security Administrator and Coordinator of Health, Welfare, and Related Defense Activities, responded by creating the National Nutrition Advisory Committee. The National Research Council appointed a Committee on Foods and Nutrition, which produced the tables of recommended daily allowances for men and women of different ages and types of work, as well as for children, and expectant and nursing mothers. State nutrition committees, county steering committees, and local action committees were also established, with the aim of carrying out a large-scale educational program aimed, not at those on relief, but at the whole population.(44)

The National Nutrition Conference for Defense, held in Washington in May, 1941, brought together leading nutritional scientists, government bureaucrats, and others. Its goal was to ensure the availability of a nutritionally adequate diet for all, using education, and enrichment of staple foods, and the supplementing of inadequate diets (via food stamps, school lunches, low cost distribution of milk, and other methods) as means to that goal. Summarizing the conference's recommendations (and echoing the president's words quoted by McNutt in opening the conference), Frank G. Boudreau, chairman of the National Research Council's Food and Nutrition Board and its Committee on Nutrition in Industry, wrote:

> As food affects the health, strength, stamina, nervous condition, morale, and mental functioning of the individual, it is vital for this country to make full use of the modern knowledge of nutrition in this emergency, not only for the armed forces, but also for industrial workers and the whole civilian population.
>
> Widespread weaknesses in our nutritional armor have been revealed by dietary surveys, selective service examinations, and the studies of the nutritional status of individuals and groups.(45)

As war approached, the research and educational activities of the 1930s, undertaken in a context of depression, hunger, and food surplus, had taken on a new significance. They were evaluated now in terms of their contribution to national defense.

A multitude of official committees and agencies became involved in the effort to ensure nutritional adequacy for the population as a whole. Their participation suggests that there was no less awareness in the American state system than the British of the importance of nutrition for the war effort. Indeed, in the extension of the state's role in organizing and controlling the nation's food supply, in the new universalism, which identified the problem as going far beyond the dependent poor, in the efforts to keep down food prices (and hence wage demands) through rationing, price controls, and subsidies, the same basic tendencies can be seen at work in both countries. When we ask how far the state was able to assert itself cohesively in translating concern about nutrition into effective control of the situation, however, a clear contrast emerges.

In the United States, as in Britain, the state became increasingly involved in regulating the production and distribution of food. But the structure and background of food administration in the United States was completely different. As we have seen, while Britain was heavily dependent upon food imports, the United States had a much larger agricultural population, proportionately as well as absolutely, and was essentially self-sufficient in most staples. Furthermore, the size, regional variation, and governmental structure of the United States contributed to creating a more complex, varied administrative pattern, less centralized and less well adapted to emergency situations.(46) Unlike Britain, the United States had never before experienced formal rationing at the retail level, and little had been done in the way of advance planning.(47)

Both countries faced shortages, but these were much less severe in the United States, where nevertheless hunger resulted in some areas like Pascagoula, Mississippi – there, supplies of meat and milk arrived in infrequent and inadequate shipments.(48) The demands of the military and of Lend-Lease (after passage of the Lend-Lease Act on March 11, 1941), as well as of an increasingly full employment domestic economy, transformed surplus into shortage and led to a widening circle of rationing.

Responsibility for rationing and for containing inflation lay mainly with the Office of Price Administration (OPA). The relative "weakness" of the American state vis-a-vis conflicting class interests is well illustrated by the difficulties and opposition that agency encountered. As the state superseded areas of private decision making, so the decisions became open and political, matters of conscious, social, and debated choice. Far from reducing conflict through intervention of the "neutral" state (the "normative umpire," as Daniel Bell calls it), (49) the effect was to translate conflict from the economic to the political sphere, and thereby to intensify it.

Thus, Polenberg describes the OPA as a locus of conflict:

> Political controversies swarmed about the OPA like so many angry insects: Each interest group scrambled to get preferential treatment; rural and urban forces clashed over food prices; opposing factions struggled for the upper hand in local rationing boards; Congress resented what it considered the arrogant exercise of power by OPA bureaucrats; and state political machines sometimes fought to prevent OPA patronage from going to congressmen.(50)

Both major parties charged that the other was trying to use the agency for partisan advantage, and Fiorello LaGuardia commented that "prohibition was but a penny-ante game in comparison with the pickings, plunder, patronage and power" that partisan control of wartime agencies would make possible.(51) Despite his suprapolitical, bureaucratic, even technocratic aspirations ("a sort of impersonal calculating machine," he once described his official self), the first price administrator, Leon Henderson, embroiled in the political controversy he had sought to avoid, resigned after a short term in late 1942, for reasons of health.(52)

As in Britain, the fear of inflation and its effects on working-class militancy were central concerns of government food policy. (By the time of the general strike of coalminers in 1943, food prices had increased, since August 1939, by more than double the percentage increase for all other cost-of-living items.)(53) The president and the OPA sought to put a ceiling on food prices while using subsidies to farmers to compensate them for increased costs or to encourage specific lines of production. In seeking powers and funds to buy, sell, or store commodities whenever doing so would help control prices or stimulate marginal production, the OPA bureaucrats modelled their approach on the British Ministry of Food. They envisaged a closely supervised economy, with very tight controls. In the United States, however, as Benedict puts it, "people (were) less ready to abandon customary free enterprise ways and less willing to submerge special group interests for the general welfare. In addition, food and price management in the United States was greatly hampered by a complex body of price legislation designed for depression conditions which the farm groups were unwilling to give up."(54)

"Free enterprise ways" notwithstanding, Benedict himself points out that in the 1930s farmers had themselves been extensively and personally subsidized through relief funds, parity payments, soil conservation payments, and below-cost credit. Nevertheless, they bitterly opposed subsidies in the context of a sellers' market.(55) They wanted prices to rise, and consumers, who could now afford it, to become used to paying more. Business and agricultural leaders argued that control of inflation should take the form of rigid wage controls, thus holding down production costs. They distrusted the Administration as being too sympathetic to labor. While the President sought to hold down wages through no-strike agreements and relieving the wage-demand pressure arising from cost-of-living increases, he could not at first impose rigid wage controls, short of a totalitarian regimentation of labor, without jeopardizing the needed redeployment of workers into war industries. Business, agriculture, and those who spoke for them in Congress were highly suspicious of this approach, and pushed throughout the war for tighter restrictions on labor and wages on the one hand, while constantly attacking and weakening the powers of the OPA to control prices through subsidies and rationing on the other. The result was a gradual tightening of wage controls (and imposition of other anti-working-class measures, such as the Smith-Connally Act), and a weakening of price controls.

In this conflict, the state at the national executive level proved not only relatively weak, but also divided. After several years of creation, merging, and liquidation of agencies concerned with feeding the nation (and allies) in wartime, responsibility was finally settled, in March-April 1943, on the War Food Administration (WFA). This agency's ability to enforce the policy of the president in the face of sectional capitalist interests was somewhat hampered by the circumstance that its head, Marvin Jones, had been a leading representative of agricultural interests in Congress, and tended to concur with the farm-state congressmen and farm organizations. Benedict describes Jones's relations with the OPA in a way highly suggestive of the divisions and weakness within the executive branch.

He did not see eye to eye with the OPA administrators and there was a lack of close contact between the two agencies, though they were supposed to reach joint decisions on food matters. In the heat of the controversy over (price) rollbacks, Jones stated that they had been announced without his knowledge or consultation, though he was supposed to have the most important powers in the food field.(56)

A growing black market, which seems to have flourished on a considerably larger scale than in Britain, reflected the relatively weak authority of the state as representative of the collective national interest. Rationing was administered by local boards, comprising prestigious business and professional people from the community. They often reflected, more than they resisted, community pressures, with a resulting lack of uniformity across the country.(57)

Meat rationing, introduced early in 1943, ran into especially stiff opposition, which well illustrates the weakness of the state's authority and its inability to impose comprehensive, rational planning and control. In an attempt to ensure uniformity (i.e., that a particular cut of meat would be the same thing in different parts of the country), the OPA sent out extraordinarily detailed directives to butchers about exactly how to cut their meat. This effort was fiercely attacked and ridiculed by the conservative press and members of Congress, who eagerly defended the small businessman against the interfering idiocies of young Washington lawyers. The then OPA director, Prentiss M. Brown, responded by reducing not only the powers of many of his staff lawyers, but their numbers too, from 2,700 to 100.(58)

A severe meat shortage developed in the winter of 1942-1943. The partial regulation of prices left various middlemen in a squeeze. Thus, packers were caught between regulated retail prices and unregulated on-the-hoof prices. But the farm bloc in Congress refused to pass a subsidies measure that would have set an administered price for meat on the hoof. Roosevelt's 1943 rollback order, restoring prices to September 1942 levels, not only increased the hostility of cattlemen, but also provided a stimulus for the black market, which absorbed an estimated 20 percent of beef production nationwide. The government took 60 percent of prime and choice cuts of beef and 80 percent of utility grades, exacerbating the domestic civilian shortage. Meanwhile, people ate horsemeat in St. Louis and Milwaukee, muskrat in San Francisco (whether or not the 200,000 pounds of it shipped there was sold as muskrat), and went short in Pascagoula. Butter also was scarce, since most butterfat was used to produce cheese for shipment overseas. As a result of the regionally partisan activities of members of Congress from butter-producing states, the cheap subsitute, margarine, was liable to a 10-cent-per-pound federal tax if artificially colored. Eleanor Roosevelt's campaign for repeal of the tax failed.(59)

As the United States became more deeply embroiled in the war, it was subject to similar tendencies to those at work in Britain, with regard to a growing state responsibility for organizing the production, distribution, and pricing of food. Certain elements in the American conjuncture, such as the economic and political importance of agriculture, or the political hostility and conservatism of Congress, were potent in limiting state autonomization because the crisis of total war was a great deal less serious and compelling for American capital. While the national administration was unable to leave the feeding of the nation to the free play of market forces, given the tremendously inflationary impact of its other war measures, it was at the same time unable to impose the same level of planning and control that was achieved in Britain. The effect of combining the impetus to state regulation with the political pressure exerted by sectional and regional interests of the more powerful agricultural capitalists was to produce the worst, or most irrational, of both "worlds." "The tendency throughout the war," as Benedict describes it, "was to straitjacket farm prices more and more, thus moving further and further from the operation of a free market and toward a planned economy, while at the same time setting up barriers to efficient operation of a planned economy."(60) the straitjacketing arose from the farmers' insistence on demands related to "parity," that is, to a relationship with the prices of other commodities that would be similar to that prevailing in 1910-1914. Such a concept was clearly incompatible with the needs of wartime planning in the 1940s.(61) The ability of agricultural interests to impose parity on the state as a guideline to farm pricing policy is an index of the comparatively low level of autonomization achieved by the American state.

Feeding the Work Force

As more and more food items came to be in short supply, the state became increasingly concerned with ensuring that the work force received adequate food at acceptable prices. This was essential both because of the connection between nutritional adequacy and productive efficiency, and also because rising food prices in combination with a tight labor market tended, in this as in other wars, to be a spur to working-class militancy. As in Britain, millions of workers in the United States ignored threats, pleas, and intimidation from the state, employers, and union bureaucrats, and went out on illegal strikes. The strike rate in the war years was far in excess of that for legal strikes in the 1930s. In 1943, 13.5 million working days were lost through strikes in the United States, a threefold increase over the previous year.(62) Even the Communist Party, whose members became the most ardent supporters of the government and the no-strike pledge after the collapse of the Hitler-Stalin pact (they attacked picket lines, and supported speed-up, state direction of labor, and the tightening of bureaucratic control of the unions) could do little to hold back rank-and-file militancy.

Roosevelt's wartime labor policy, like that of the British government, was to encourage national labor leaders to enforce a no-strike pledge while facilitating the growth of union membership. Its aim was to convert the militant organizers of yesterday into the policers of class collaboration today. But the maintenance of political and economic stability, as well as of productivity, also required specific attention to food control. The administration responded to this need both through its rationing and price policies and through its encouragement of industrial feeding facilities.

Those who were fit enough to be inducted into the armed forces naturally received the best available diet, one that was planned by the military's nutritionists to be balanced and sufficient, and one that was provided at state expense. The war worker's situation was different. "Huge new plants, located away from built-up communities, with little or no provision for feeding the workers, place almost insuperable obstacles in the way of good nutrition," complained Boudreau, adding that the National Research Council's Committee on Nutrition in Industry was organizing controlled studies to discover the effects of improved nutrition of defense workers on absenteeism, accidents, and production.(63)

The OPA's General Maximum Price Regulation of April 28, 1942 froze prices on about 60 percent of all civilian food items, and ration books based on a point system were issued to all. Sugar and coffee were first to be rationed, but they were followed by meats, butter and other fats, and canned goods. Much of the food shortage in the United States resulted from the diversion of supplies to meet the needs of the armed forces and of allies. It was a great deal less serious than in other major combatant countries, including Britain.

The American government, like the British, rejected the systematic use of differential rationing, of the kind that was in force in Germany. Under such a system, individuals received different allowances or ration points according to their occupation or some other criterion. Special treatment was afforded certain groups, nevertheless, and many more groups in Britain than in the United States. Infants, children under five years, and industrial workers, all received favored treatment of some kind in Britain. There was much less differential rationing of any kind in the United States, but supplemental allowances were made for invalids and for certain isolated groups of workers like lumberjacks and seamen. In part this difference may reflect the less complete and detailed regulation of social and economic life by the American state than the British (or German). In part it simply reflects the fact that rationing was much less stringent in the United States, so that differential rationing, direct or indirect, was less necessary to prevent hardship to groups with special needs.(64)

The war, it has been noted, represented much less of a threat to American capital than to British. In consequence, it required a lower (though still high) level of mobilization of the whole population, and so required fewer concessions to them. The provision of extra rations for certain groups of workers came late in the war, and not before a number of strikes in which the availability of adequate food was an issue. In this area as in others, the American state, especially in contrast with the British, appears less as taking the initiative in a comprehensive response to a perceived problem than as reacting in an ad hoc manner to particular points of pressure from below.

Meat rationing was controversial among workers as well as those controlling its production. The ration, while a third more than that in Britain, did not allow for the special needs (and habits) of certain groups of workers engaged in heavy work and unable to obtain adequate substitutes. The issue was forced on the government's notice by the militancy of these groups, in particular loggers and miners. In the southwestern Pennsylvania coalfield, before the 1943 strike, a visiting reporter observed that:

> The most conservative miners as well as the most radical ones anticipate a slow-up, serious disturbances or possibly a rapidly spreading general strike unless positive and reliable assurances as to the food supply are given them at once.(65)

While shortages were the main concern of the miners ("A man couldn't do the work if he only had lettuce sandwiches in his lunch pail"), (66) food prices exacerbated the problem and strengthened the demand for higher wages. Food prices had risen 44 percent since the miners' last raise of $1 a day in 1941; the food comprised nearly 40 percent of their budget. In Wyoming, miners threatened to strike unless they were guaranteed seven pounds of meat a week each.(67)

Lumberjacks also protested their meat ration, and in the state of Washington, struck for higher meat rations in 1943. Wartime had produced a greatly increased demand for timber and wood pulp, and at the same time led to a labor shortage, as many lumberjacks left the forests for the defense industries. The War Food Administration (WFA) responded to this situation by conducting a study in four logging camps, in the spring of 1943, to discover the habitual food consumption patterns of lumberjacks. The WFA then requested the Food and Nutrition Board of the National Research Council to study the caloric requirements of industrial workers. The board recommended a division into four categories according to the caloric requirements of different occupations. Loggers were alone in the top category. Miners, along with foundry workers, construction workers, and longshoremen and stevedores, were in Category II. These recommendations, with slight modification, became the basis for all subsequent actions by the WFA and OPA in supplying extra amounts of food to workers in heavy industries.(68)

On May 1, 1944, loggers became the first group to receive extra rations. They were followed, in the first half of 1945, by deep-sea fishermen, and some other groups, as well as by isolated construction workers, railroad maintenance workers, and miners, where these workers ate in employee feeding establishments. Since on-the-job feeding was very rare in the mining industry, the OPA granted supplemental rations to miners individually, in the final months of the war.(69)

In reviewing and confirming its earlier recommendations, the Food and Nutrition Board's Committee on the Nutrition of Industrial Workers observed that:

> Workers engaged in activities requiring a large expenditure of energy cannot be expected to continue such activities over any period of time unless they are supplied with an adequate amount of food. If the amount of energy they obtain in the form of food is diminished, it is to be expected that they will expend less energy, i.e., do less work.(70)

Recognition of the social policy implications of capital's need for an adequate supply of efficient labor power required some prompting from below, in the form of pressure exerted by loggers, miners, and others for decent standards of health and nutrition.

For industrial workers in general, there was no American equivalent of the British Restaurants, by which they could receive additional food cheaply and off the ration from state-run facilities. There was no requirement that employers provide workplace cafeterias or canteens. Nevertheless, relying upon the voluntary cooperation of management and labor, the government did take an active interest in the nutrition of workers in industry during World War II, especially in the area of workplace feeding.*

The WFA offered technical advice about industrial feeding to management and labor, and to other federal, state, and local

---

*A Nutrition Policy and Planning Committee was created in August 1940, which in November of the same year became the Nutrition Advisory Committee to the coordinator of Health, Welfare, and Related Defense Activities. In August 1942, a Nutrition in Industry Section was established within the Nutrition Division of the Office of Defense, Health and Welfare Services, but responsibility was transferred to the WFA, where it remained from its creation in March 1943 to its termination in June 1945. To formalize the various cooperative arrangements that developed between the WFA and other federal agencies, another organization was established in October 1943, the Inter-Agency Committee on Food for Workers (International Labour Office, Nutrition in Industry, pp. 54-58).

agencies and groups. It was mainly responsible for nutrition education programs, and solely responsible for solving food supply problems involving nonrationed items. The agency had no power to enforce its recommendations about in-plant feeding facilities or nutrition education programs, except that, from April 1944, it had and used the authority to certify as to the appropriateness of floor plans and the adequacy of facilities for industrial food services. On this certification depended the possibility of the War Production Board's granting priorities that would permit installation.(71)

While in-plant feeding was common before World War II, it expanded greatly during the war, and improved considerably in terms of food service facilities, food preparation, and service. Comparison of the survey conducted by the National Association of Manufacturers in 1940 with the WFA's 1944 survey indicates that about 65 percent of the workers employed in manufacturing plants had food service facilities in 1940, compared with 81 percent of those in 1944.(72) The percentage of plants with food services increased from 41 percent to 49 percent, the probability (in both surveys) increasing with plant size (see Table 3). The figures do not accurately reflect the great expansion in industrial feeding that took place during the war. Not only is the percentage increase of workers in plants with feeding facilities much greater than the percentage increase of plants with such provision, but the number of workers in manufacturing plants increased enormously, from 7.8 million in 1939 to 16.5 million in 1944.(73) Of course, not all workers used the cafeteria or other feeding facilities. While, in 1944, four out of five war workers in manufacturing were in plants with food service facilities, only 38.5 percent actually obtained meals from them.(74)

It is likely that in-plant feeding would have expanded and improved in World War II, even without the stimulus and assistance of the WFA. The scarcity of labor, the location of many war-industry plants, and the uprooted or migrant character of much of the work force (many living in lodgings with no cooking facilities) give reason to think so. It is also true that many other government activities had an impact upon the nutritional status of workers, including the OPA's control of prices and the bread and flour enrichment program. But the WFA (especially its Industrial Feeding Programs Division) undoubtedly played an important role. Its team of Industrial Feeding specialists gave much advice and assistance on facilities, operating problems, and nutrition education programs. They also produced many practical, informational publications, and conducted many studies, of dietary habits, of the impact of nutrition education programs, of absenteeism and disability.

Because in the United States, unlike Britain, the feeding of workers on the job was essentially a matter of management choice, there was wide variation between plants, in the presence or absence of a cafeteria, in the atmosphere, the quality of the food, and the extent to which it was subsidized by the corporation. The state, in the form of the WFA, did not require provision or guarantee minimum standards in this area, but was limited to a facilitating role. In its reliance upon official encouragement rather than governmental compulsion and control, American industrial feeding policy in World War II more closely resembled the British approach in the first World War than in the second. It is, then, not the state of nutritional science (which was the same in both countries) that we must look for an explanation of policy differences, but to the kind of pressures, threats, or vulnerabilities, internal and external, to which the state was obliged to respond. In this respect, it should be reemphasized that the United States, like Britain in the 1914-1918 War, faced a less dangerous military threat, suffered less disruption of industrial life (and civilian life in general), and had a less acute labor shortage than Britain in the second World War.

TABLE 3
Percentage of Manufacturing Plants with Food Services

Plant Employment Size	NAM Survey (1940)	WFA Survey (1944)
All sizes	41	49
1-249	25	28
250-499	37	46
500-999	50	63
1,000-1,999	65	--
1,000-2,499	--	80
2,000-over	77	--
2,500-over	--	91

Source: International Labour Office, Nutrition in Industry, p. 61.

Welfare Food Programs

In the United States, as in Britain, the national government became involved in the 1930s in a number of welfare food programs, but on a larger scale. These were aimed selectively at the poor, and were shaped by the existence of a large agricultural surplus and, especially in the case of the school lunch program, designed to provide work relief. In Britain, we have seen, the welfare food programs were expanded in World War II, developing in a universalist direction to take in all members of priority groups. With the decline of employment and food surpluses in the United States, on the other hand, the major welfare food programs of the federal government, notably commodity distribution and food stamps, were cut back almost to nothing or eliminated altogether. The main exception was the school lunch program, which was discontinued in its existing form (involving direct distribution through state welfare agencies of federally purchased surplus foods), but was replaced on a more permanent basis not contingent upon the existence of surpluses.

The food stamp program was suspended in March, 1943. Surplus commodity distribution was discontinued in the same year, and most of the local distribution machinery dismantled, though some revival took place as surpluses materialized again in a few areas. "With the disappearance of surpluses and the decrease in public assistance cases," reported the secretary of agriculture in 1943, "the direct distribution, food stamps, and other governmental programs through which foods were made available to needy consumers have been discontinued."(75) Other factors no doubt played a role too, such as concern about irregularities in implementation of the food stamp plan at the retail level, and doubts about the program's efficacy as a means of increasing overall demand for agricultural produce.(76) Nevertheless, these programs were from their inception tied to the existence of an agricultural surplus, and disappeared with little fuss when the surplus was replaced by shortage. A national food allotment plan, by which any family would have been able to exchange a specified percentage of its income, say 40 percent, for stamps sufficient to purchase an adequate minimum diet, was much discussed in the Senate Committee on Agriculture and Forestry as part of a postwar policy for agriculture, but was never passed by Congress.(77)

Among the welfare food programs to be discontinued in 1943 was that for subsidizing the sale of milk to needy families. In effect from 1939 to 1943, like the food stamp plan, it operated on a much more modest scale, expenditures peaking at under $4 million in 1941-1942 compared with $115.8 million in 1942 for food stamps. While the "penny milk" part of the milk subsidy became fused with the school lunch program, and survived with it, the relief milk distributed to needy families (through an indemnity for handlers who sold it at a special low price) was discontinued in 1943, because of the decrease in public assistance cases and the shortage of milk.(78)

In Britain, we have seen, the same factors – decline of welfare rolls and appearance of food shortages – were at work, but a considerable expansion, and extension beyond the poor, of subsidized milk and other welfare food programs, nevertheless took place. The official response there was not that there was no surplus milk to give away, but that, given a shortage of milk, the limited supply should go first to those who needed it, regardless of their ability to pay. Priority groups were given first preference on the available supply, and subsidized in their purchase of it. The reasons for this more rational-comprehensive approach of the British state, for its greater degree of autonomy, have been suggested in the previous chapter.

When the state's interest in the health of the population is extended by war beyond the military, Titmuss suggests in his "War and Social Policy" essay, it is directed first at school children, the next generation of recruits.(79) Certainly it was the welfare food programs for American school children, the school lunch and milk programs, which survived and were freed from dependence upon an agricultural surplus. The war both jeopardized the development of the 1930s in school feeding, and stimulated progress in the direction of a permanent program.

In 1942, California Representative Jerry Voorhis, prompted by the draft rejection rates, made the first legislative attempt to earmark federal funds specifically for a national school lunch program. The attempt failed.

By 1943, the basis of federal involvement in the school lunch programs was eliminated. In a time of mass unemployment it was a useful source of work relief jobs, but with a scarce labor supply and the abolition of the WPA, the school food services were deprived of a valuable pool of trained employees. Full employment also expanded demand for food, while large quantities were required for the armed forces and for allies under Lend-Lease. By 1943 the food surpluses drawn upon by the school lunch programs had largely disappeared. While the schools had received a peak of 454.5 million pounds of surplus commodities in the 1941-1942 school year, by 1943 the supply was limited almost entirely to eggs, fresh fruit, and vegetables.(80)

The future of the program was in doubt. In 1943 the Food Distribution Administration of the WFA received congressional approval of a plan to support school lunch programs through a cash indemnity of $50 million, earmarked for this purpose in the Agricultural Appropriation Act. Under this scheme, schools and others running nonprofit school lunch programs bought certain foods locally and were reimbursed at a specific rate, according to the type of meals served. The appropriation was for the fiscal year ending June 30, 1944, and no provision was made for federal assistance after that date.(81)

An attempt was made to amend the (1944) Agriculture Appropriation bill, earmarking $50 million for federal participation in the school lunch program. The House of Representatives voted it down, 136 to 54, on March 7, 1944. Federal funding for school lunches was thereby eliminated. While liberals like Voorhis (California), Murdock (Arizona), and Sabath (Illinois) spoke for the amendment, it was strongly opposed on several grounds. Opponents argued that the federal government was already deeply in debt and becoming more so, whereas state and local governments (whose responsibility school lunches rightly were anyway) were experiencing diminishing indebtedness and so were in better position to finance the program. Furthermore, most citizens were "enjoying great prosperity," and parents could, and should, provide for their own children. Rep.

Hoffman (Michigan) saw the program as just another attempt to make "sissies and panty-waists" of American children.(82)

The advocates of a national school lunch program did not give up. In April 1944, the Committee to Obtain the Support of Congress for a Nationwide School Lunch Program (a joint committee of the National School Cafetaria Association and the Food Service Directors' Conference) distributed a statement to 30,000 schools "in which it depicted the school lunch program not only as an organized effort to feed the hungry but as a means of ensuring the physical vigor of the youth of America so that they might enjoy individual success and meet the 'imperative needs of our country' in times of danger."(83) In the same month three bills were introduced in the Senate to continue federal assistance for school lunches. In May the Pace bill (HR 4268), originating in and approved by the House, was amended by the Senate Agriculture Committee to include federal assistance for school lunches under the WFA. In June the bill, which provided for continuation of federal funding for two years, was approved in conference. The result was that Congress authorized a specific amount of funds for the operation of the school lunch and penny-milk programs and provided for the carrying out of these activities regardless of the existence of a food surplus.(84) Two years later, in June 1946, the National School Lunch Act, establishing a permanent, conditional grant-in-aid program, became law. The conditions were that the programs must be nonprofit, meet nutritional standards, provide free or reduced price lunches for needy pupils without discrimination, and account for their funds to the federal government. Within these guidelines, the state and local school officials would control operation of the program.(85)

Federal involvement in school lunches, then, followed a pattern similar to that of the school meals service in Britain, though it was not to become as extensive. From an emphasis on feeding the destitute and absorbing surplus food in the 1930s, the program shifted in wartime to safeguarding the nation's children by serving nutritious meals and developing good food habits.

The survival and expansion of the school lunch program may be understood in terms of the kind of functional explanation offered by Titmuss for the early (relative to other population groups) development of the state's concern for the health of school children. Such an account would be incomplete, however, if it did not recognize the greater legitimacy and more powerful constituency enjoyed by this program, compared with the other welfare food programs. School administrators had long sought control of the program, emphasizing its educational purposes. They believed that federal funds should be administered by the Office of Education rather than the Department of Agriculture. But they argued strongly for the continuation of a school lunch program, regardless of its utility for agriculture. Nutritional and educational goals were, indeed, more evident, and seemed more clearly realized in this than in other welfare food programs, a fact that enhanced its legitimacy. Furthermore, school lunches had been served prior to and independently of the availability of surplus commodities, and not only to the poor. Though the federal government, by offering surplus food and surplus labor, had sought to assist and extend school lunch facilities, they had existed, and would continue to do so on some scale, even without that assistance. The school lunch program, then, had more of a base, and more legitimacy, than the other welfare food programs.

CONCLUSION

In response to the crisis of World War II, the American state took measures to protect the nutritional status of the population (and certain sections in particular, such as the armed forces, industrial workers, school children) that were in many respects similar to those taken by the British. In the United States, however, the state went less far in organizing the allocation of food (rationing and price control), in safeguarding the position of specific groups, and in shifting social welfare provision in a universalist direction.

The state, at national executive level, ran into more vigorous and effective opposition to the extension of its power and the assertion of its relative autonomy — from legislators reflecting regional or sectional capitalist interests (especially agriculture), from conservative legislators opposed on principle to such extension and assertion, and from particular sectors of capital (e.g., the meat industry) who were relatively successful in defending their specific interests against federal government attempts to subordinate them to more general capitalist interests.

If resistance to the state was stronger in the United States, it could afford to be so because the internal and external threats were weaker. The need for an adequate supply of efficient industrial and military manpower, as well as for national solidarity, was certainly made more pressing by the war. It was impressed on the state and capital by such factors as the draft rejection rates, the rising tempo of workplace struggle (including strikes in which food-related demands were prominent), and the example of British food control. But neither pressures like these nor the direct military threat of the war itself had as strongly coercive a force as in Britain.

NOTES

(1)   John A. Garraty, "New Deal, National Socialism, and Great Depression," pp. 907-44. For a brief but suggestive comparison of the British and American experience of the Depression, see Jim Potter, The American Economy Between the World Wars, pp. 100-1.

(2)   Richard Osborn Cummings, American and His Food, pp. 177-80; Edwin G. Nourse, Marketing Agreements, passim.

(3)   Cummings, American and His Food, pp. 188-89; Harry Hopkins, Spending to Save, pp. 154-56; Josephine C. Brown, Public Relief, p. 254; U. S. FERA Monthly Report, July 1935.

(4)   Cummings, American, p. 189.

(5)   Elmer V. McCollum, Newer Knowledge of Nutrition. Todhunter observes that the expansion of McCollum's book, from 189 pages in its first edition (1918) to 684 pages in its fifth (1939), reflects the rapid growth of nutritional knowledge in this period. Todhunter, "Story of Nutrition," p. 12.

(6)   Brown, Public Relief, pp. 74-75.

(7)   Cummings, American, p. 188.

(8)   John Donald Black and Maxine Enlow Kiefer, Future Food and Agriculture Policy, pp. 1, 26.

(9)   See U. S. Federal Security Agency, National Nutrition Conference, pp. 10, 31; Gove Hambidge, "Nutrition as a National Problem," p. 362. See also Chapter 3, n. 8.

(10)   Benedict, Farm Policies, p. 385.

(11)   Ibid.

(12)   Ibid.

(13)   Miriam Birdseye, Extension Work.

(14   Gladys Lucille Baker, The County Agent, p. 93.

(15)   Ibid.

(16)   George Rosen, History of Public Health, pp. 416-17; Sophia Halsted, "The Nutritionist in a City Public Health Program," pp. 850-51; Marjorie Heseltine, "Nutrition Services in Maternal and Child Health," pp. 814-16; Heseltine, "The Nutritionist's Place," pp. 167-69; Mary A. Mason, "Food and Nutrition in the FERA," pp. 223-24.

(17)   Arguments questioning the adequacy of educational efforts alone, or claiming that low purchasing power was the primary cause of malnutrition, were made by Heseltine, "The Nutritionist's Place," p. 167; Virginia Britton, "The Cost of Food," pp. 294-96; Hambidge, "Nutrition as a National Problem," pp. 361-64; Helen L. Sorenson and Elizabeth W. Gilboy, "Economics of Low Income Diets," pp. 663-80; Edwin G. Nourse, "Economic Problem of Nutrition," p. 341; T. Swain Harding, "America's Food Problem," pp. 209-10; Emily White Stevens, "Is There Too Much Food?" pp. 297-99. For arguments in favor of an educational emphasis in dealing with malnutrition, see Ellery F. Reed, Need of Casework, p. 6; Morris Fishbein, National Nutrition, pp. 12, 188, passim.

(18)   Fishbein, National Nutrition, p. 199.

(19)   Cummings, American and His Food, pp. 204-05; Margaret G. Reid, Consumers and the Market, p. 543.

(20)   Josephine C. Brown, Public Relief, p. 226.

(21)   Ibid, p. 227.

(22)   Ibid, pp. 242-44; see also Joanna C. Colcord, Cash Relief.

(23)   Brown, Public Relief, p. 255.

(24)   Howard P. Davis, "Sharing Our Bounty," p. 688.

(25)   Benedict, Farm Policies, p. 381.

(26)   Thelma G. Flanagan, "School Food Services," p. 562; Cummings, American, p. 198.

(27)   Cummings, American, pp. 219-20.

(28)   Martha Branscombe, "Reports From the Food Stamp Front," pp. 341-43; Colcord, "Stamps," pp. 305-7.

(29)   Joseph D. Coppock, "Food Stamp Plan"; Don Paarlberg, Subsidized Food Consumption, pp. 44-45; Kenneth W. Clarkson, Food Stamps and Nutrition.

(30)   Marvin M. Sandstrom, "School Lunches," p. 692.

(31)   Ibid., p. 693.

(32)   Flanagan, "School Food Services," p. 561.

(33)   Ibid., pp. 561-62.

(34)   Sandstrom, School Lunches, p. 694. Cf. Paarlberg, Subsidized Food Consumption, p. 29; Cummings, American, p. 216.

(35)   Flanagan, "School Food Services," p. 563; U. S. Department of Agriculture, Report of Secretary, 1940, p. 54.

(36)   USDA, Report of Secretary, p. 54.

(37)   Alan S. Milward, War, Economy and Society, p. 272; Benedict, Farm Policies, p. 400.

(38)   Benedict, Farm Policies, p. 402.

(39)   Ibid., p. 351. See also Hugh H. Bennett, Soil Conservation; Charles M. Hardin, Politics of Agriculture; Edgar B. Nixon, ed., Roosevelt and Conservation.

(40)   U. S. Federal Security Agency, National Nutrition Conference, pp. 63-67.

(41)   George W. Bachman and Lewis Meriam, Compulsory Health Insurance, pp. 6, 22-23, 111-20.

(42)   U. S. Senate, Committee on Education and Labor, Subcommittee on Health and Education, Wartime Health, p. 602.

(43)   Survey Midmonthly 84 (August 1944): 235.

(44)   Cummings, American, pp. 231-39.

(45)   Frank G. Boudreau, "Food for a Vital America," p. 129.

(46)   Eric Roll, Combined Food Board, p. 8.

(47)   William A. Nielander, Wartime Food Rationing, pp. 113, 115.

(48)   U. S. Senate, Committee on Education and Labor, Wartime Health, Part 2, pp. 945-1004. See also Janeway, Struggle for Survival.

(49)   Daniel Bell, "Public Household," pp. 37-38.

(50)   Richard Polenberg, War and Society, p. 33.

(51)   LaGuardia to Prentiss M. Brown, April 21, 1943, Roosevelt Papers, OF4403. Cited by Polenberg, War and Society, p. 33.

(52)   Polenberg, War and Society, pp. 33-34.

(53)   Benedict, Farm Policies, p. 426.

(54)   Ibid., p. 419. Cf. p. 410. See also James S. Earley, L. Margaret Hall, and Marjorie S. Berger, British Wartime Price Administration, 1939-1943, Office of Price Administration, February 10, 1944.

(55)   Benedict, Farm Policies, p. 419.
(56)   Ibid., p. 427, n. 77.
(57)   Polenberg, War and Society, pp. 32-33.
(58)   Richard R. Lingeman, Don't You Know There's a War On? pp. 312-13.
(59)   Ibid., pp. 314-17; Benedict, Farm Policies, pp. 402-30; U. S. Senate, Committee on Education and Labor, Wartime Health, Part 2, pp. 995-1004 et passim.
(60)   Benedict, Farm Policies, p. 417.
(61)   Benedict, Can We Solve? p. 13; idem. Farm Policies, pp. 416-17 et passim.
(62)   Alan Milward, War, Economy, and Society, p. 243; Joel Seidman, American Labor from Defense to Reconversion, pp. 275-76. For a valuable collection of radical essays on relations among state, employers, union bureaucrats, and rank-and-file workers, see the special issue of Radical America, "American Labor in the 1940's," 9, nos. 4-5 (1975).
(63)   Boudreau, "Food for a Vital America," p. 156.
(64)   Nielander, Wartime Food Rationing, pp. 128-30.
(65)   Agnes E. Meyer, Journey Through Chaos, p. 230.
(66)   John Dos Passos, State of the Nation, p. 234.
(67)   Lingeman, Don't You Know? pp. 317-18.
(68)   International Labour Office, Nutrition in Industry, pp. 89-91.
(69)   Ibid., pp. 94-95.
(70)   U. S. National Research Council, Proceedings of the Food and Nutrition Board 5 (Sept. 26, 1945): 140.
(71)   International Labour Office, Nutrition in Industry, p. 58.
(72)   National Association of Manufacturers, Industrial Health Practices; U. S. Department of Agriculture, Industrial Feeding.
(73)   International Labour Office, Nutrition in Industry, p. 61.
(74)   Ibid., p. 64.
(75)   USDA, Report of Secretary, 1943, p. 63.
(76)   See Leon Gold, A. C. Hoffman, Frederick V. Waugh, Economic Analysis of Food Stamp Plan; Coppock, "Food Stamp Plan."
(77)   Benedict, Can We Solve?, p. 290.
(78)   Herman M. Southworth, "Economics of Public Measures to Subsidize Food Consumption," p. 43.
(79)   Richard M. Titmuss, "War and Social Policy," p. 80.
(80)   Flanagan, "School Food Services," p. 564.
(81)   Catherine T. Long, "School Lunch Legislation," p. 258.
(82)   Ibid. Survey Midmonthly 80 (April 1944): 128; Newsweek (April 17, 1944): 105-6; Geoffrey Perrett, Days of Sadness, p. 328.
(83)   Flanagan, "School Food Services," p. 565.
(84)   Long, "School Lunch Legislation," p. 258; Survey Midmonthly 80 (April 1944): 128; Sandstrom, "School Lunches," p. 694.
(85)   Flanagan, "School Food Services," p. 566.

6

TUBERCULOSIS CONTROL
IN WARTIME

Even in the midst of war, one cannot afford to ignore an enemy which kills 25,000 people every year in this country and is still, except for war and accidents, the chief destroyer of man and woman-power in its prime.(1)

The British minister of health, who used those words at a press conference about the new tuberculosis allowances scheme in 1943, might more accurately have said that "especially" rather than "even" in the midst of war tuberculosis could not be ignored. As a disease whose incidence and mortality rates tended to increase in wartime, and one that threatened to worsen still further the desperate shortage of military and industrial manpower, tuberculosis commanded a new level of state response from both British and American governments. At the same time, as the British experience revealed, two narrow a focus on manpower and wartime emergency needs led to contradictions in program design and problems of legitimation.

War, we have seen, increased the state's involvement in efforts to protect and improve the nutritional status of the population. But, as Chapter 3 emphasized, actual levels of nutrition were a function not only of food and nutrition policy, but also a more or less unintended side effect of other aspect of government policy and of nonpolicy economic and social developments. Deliberate nutrition policy, on the other hand, may in some respects have been counterproductive. Similar considerations apply in the case of tuberculosis, in part because nutrition itself was an especially important determinant of the disease's incidence. (Nutrition powerfully affected resistance to the disease, while the other key determinant, overcrowding, produced more or less heavy exposure to it.) The focus on

92

mass radiography and other screening and case-finding efforts, on exclusion (or incentives for withdrawal) from the work force and military, and on rehabilitation reflects the direction of deliberate state activity, in Britain and the United States, to control tuberculosis. It does not, of course, imply that these measures were the prime agents of the disease's more or less continued decline.

THE PREWAR BACKGROUND

Britain

Tuberculosis, the "white plague," was the "captain of all the men of death" (2) in nineteenth century Britain. Rather than striking in short, sharp epidemics like typhoid or smallpox, it was continuously present. It attacked men and women in their most productive years, claiming victims from all social classes, but especially from the poor, overcrowded unsanitary working-class sections of the industrial cities.

In the last part of the century, however, even before the discovery of the tubercle baccilus in 1882, and before the antituberculosis movement had made much impact, tuberculosis retreated in the face of improvements in sanitation, nutrition, real wages, working conditions, housing, and other aspects of the general standard of life. By the turn of the century it had given way, as the nation's leading fatal disease, to influenza and pneumonia. Its decline continued during the twentieth centry, except for a very sharp rise during World War I.(3)* The medical advances of the 1880s and 1890s, however, including not only the discovery of the tubercle baccilus, but also the elaboration of the germ theory of disease in general, gave impetus to an international antituberculosis movement, incorporating and extending the new medical and public health approaches to disease control. In the first decade of the twentieth century, tuberculosis no longer seemed inevitable. Aggressive state intervention to control the disease and help its victims became, as never before, a credible policy option.

The last Liberal government, stimulated both by the the concern, arising from the Boer War, about the "physical deterioration" of the

*"Tuberculosis was, in effect," René Dubos observes, "the social disease of the nineteenth century, perhaps the first penalty that capitalistic society had to pay for the ruthless exploitation of labor" (White Plague, p. 207). Many epidemics, including tuberculosis, reach a peak "shortly after the shift from a rural to an industrial type of economy; then the epidemics lose their acute character and their mortality falls as prosperity becomes more widespread" (Mirage of Health, p. 194). Wars and upheavals interrupt the decline (White Plague, pp. 194-96).

population and by the rising independence and militancy of the labor movement, enacted far-reaching reforms in health and welfare. One product of this legislation, in the context of the new medical and public health understanding of the disease, was a great expansion of the state's role in measures dealing with tuberculosis. The first step was to require that those treating tuberculous patients notify the public health authorities of all their cases. Public health regulations of 1908, 1911, and 1912 extended the requirement of notification first to cases under the care of Poor Law medical officers, then to all cases treated by hospitals, dispensaries, or sanatoria, then to all cases of pulmonary tuberculosis under medical care, and finally to cover all forms of tuberculosis.(4)

By 1912, then, notification was compulsory. Treatment facilities were limited, however, largely to beds in voluntary and Poor Law general hospitals, and to a few sanatoria and dispensaries. There was a considerable overall shortage.(5) the National Insurance Act of 1911 addressed the tuberculosis problem by including treatment of the disease as a benefit, by providing for reasearch and education, and by promising funds for sanatoria and other facilities. These provisions reflected both Lloyd George's concern for the national health and, more specifically, the fear that tuberculosis would swamp the new insurance scheme to the point of threatening its financial soundness, if stronger measures were not taken to control the disease.(6)

Waldorf Astor, a "Tory who believed in social reform and a Christian Scientist who favored medical research,"(7) played an important role in developing the tuberculosis provisions of the 1911 National Insurance Act. He became chairman of the Departmental Committee on Tuberculosis, which was set up in the wake of the act in February 1912. The Astor Report, produced by this committee, laid down the lines on which the tuberculosis service would be established, and on which it still ran in the 1930s. Central government provided matching funds to local authorities for the operation of the service, as well as capital grants for treatment facilities. The tuberculosis service was a matter for each locality to organize, as part of its public health administration.(8)

The plan proposed by Astor, and mandated for local authorities by the Public Health (Tuberculosis) Act of 1921, involved at the first level the tuberculosis dispensary. A center for diagnosis, case finding, and some forms of treatment, as well as for education and aftercare, the dispensary acted as a clearing house. Its specialist medical staff (tuberculosis officers, supported by tuberculosis visitors and nurses) visited homes, examined contacts, and referred patients for residential treatment.

At the second level were the sanatoria, hospitals, and other residential facilities. Even before the Great War of 1914-1918, there were not enough of them to meet the demand. The war, accompanied by increased industrialization, the physical and emotional stress of war, long work hours, and overcrowding, produced a sharp rise in mortality from tuberculosis. While increasing the relative shortage of beds, it stimulated efforts for more comprehensive national responsibility for health, one outcome of which was the establishment of the Ministry of Health in 1919.

Provision of more beds was, then, an early priority of the tuberculosis service. The number increased substantially following the first World War, and again in the 1930s, when the Local Government Act of 1929 enabled local authorities to appropriate poor law institutions, or parts of them, for use as tuberculosis hospitals.(9)

By the end of 1937, when the planning group, PEP (Political and Economic Planning), published its report on the British health services, tuberculosis was still accounting for more deaths among the 10-40 age group than any other disease. Nearly half of all deaths of women between 20 and 25 years of age were due to tuberculosis. For men and women the risk of contracting pulmonary tuberculosis was highest in the early twenties. It declined rapidly with increasing age for women, but reached a secondary peak for men at about 50 years, the age at which most male deaths from the disease occurred. The effects of urbanization were found to be strongest for men over 45 years, while within cities tuberculosis was associated with poverty and overcrowding.(10) Working men and women in the industrial cities were the people hardest hit by the disease, and they were most likely to succumb to it in their productive years. Loss of manpower would be a serious problem to the state in wartime (there were 230,000 active or recently active cases under supervision by English, Welsh, and Scottish dispensaries in 1938),(11) and the problem was exacerbated by the chronic, slow-developing nature of the disease. Breadwinners were reluctant to disclose their illness, perhaps even to themselves, or to seek medical help, when their livelihoods were likely to be jeopardized. Staying at work, they increased the risk of infection to others. The scale of the problem is suggested by the finding that almost 10 percent of deaths from tuberculosis in England in 1936 were cases that had never been reported to the government.(12) (René and Jean Dubos put the figure for large American cities as high as 30 percent).(13) Social policy would have to address the problem of keeping as many such cases as possible out of the work force when war raised prices for the families and created an acute labor shortage for employers. It was the opposite of the problem to which "less eligibility" had been the New Poor Law's solution.

The distribution and quality of the tuberculosis services were very uneven. Under relatively weak central control and supervision, more than 150 separate authorities operated their own programs. In this fragmented response to the problem of tuberculosis, voluntary bodies played an important role. They organized care committees (though these were sometimes run by local authorities), which provided aftercare and advice, and sometimes food, clothing, or emergency financial assistance. "Approved dispensaries" supplied outpatient treatment under voluntary as well as public auspices. Voluntary bodies also maintained more than a quarter of the beds for the tuberculous (the remainder being in local authority facilities) and a small number of "village settlements." The National Association for the Prevention of Tuberculosis, founded in 1898, carried on educational and publicity work, and ran a "colony" for tuberculous boys.(14)

Another sphere of antituberculosis activity was control of the disease in cattle, which had a very high rate of infection in Britain and were responsible for much disease in people. The government regulated the milk supply in part as a way to control tuberculosis. Its efforts at eradicating bovine tuberculosis were neither as drastic nor as successful as in the United States, however, and it was estimated that 80 percent of abdominal tuberculosis, 35 percent of bone and joint disease, and 64 percent of cervical gland infections were of bovine origin.(15) Before the war about 40 percent of cattle reacted to the tuberculin test, a similar proportion slaughtered in abattoirs were found to be tuberculous, and one milk cow in every 200 had tuberculosis of the udder and was excreting virulent tubercle bacilli in its milk.(16)

Tuberculosis rates, it was increasingly acknowledged, were a function of the quality of life in general. In the absence of a vaccine recognized as being both safe and effective,* and of any specific treatment, disease control depended heavily upon more far-reaching improvements in social arrangements and living standards. Policy makers and planners understood the link between tuberculosis and nutrition in the 1930s (a link highlighted in a study by Boyd Orr and J. L. Gilks in 1931),(17) as well as other aspects of the pathogenic environment to which "cured" patients often returned. Despite an increasing state role in controlling the disease, however, the official response was still a fragmented and uneven series of initiatives, rather than a comprehensive attack.

United States

As in Britain and for the same reasons, mortality from tuberculosis was already declining in the United States before the application of the medical discoveries of the 1880s and 1890s, and before the emergence of the antituberculosis movement in the first decade of the twentieth century. Here, too, the disease struck those

---

*BCG, a vaccine developed in the 1920s and used extensively in Scandinavia and some other European countries, never gained wide acceptance in Britain or the United States.

in their most productive years, and hit the poor in the industrial cities hardest. Racial minorities were especially susceptible.(18)

Efforts at control followed a similar pattern to that in Britain. Notification, or reporting, was an early focus of reformers' efforts, and in the first decade of the century many states passed laws requiring physicians to report all cases of tuberculosis. The National Association for the Study and Prevention of Tuberculosis (later the National Tuberculosis Association), founded in 1904 and comprising both medical and lay people, carried on extensive educational, promotional, and advisory activities.(19) Other voluntary organizations also contributed to the antituberculosis movement. Both New York's Charity Organization Society (in 1902) and the New York State Aid Association (in 1907) set up Committees on the Prevention of Tuberculosis. An international conference on tuberculosis, held in Washington, D.C., in 1908, convinced reformers of the importance of residential treatment both for the provision of proper care and to reduce the risk of spreading the disease to others. The most influential proponent of this view was Arthur Newsholme, chief medical officer of the British Local Government Board.(20)

But the compulsory case reporting and increased emphasis on hospitalization brought out clearly the great shortage of beds for the tuberculous and the inadequacy of voluntary and private resources. State laws usually provided appropriations for the setting up of tuberculosis hospitals. By 1923, only three states (Nevada, New Mexico, and Wyoming) had no laws relating to tuberculosis, and of the others only two did not make provisions for hospital treatment.(21) By 1928, three quarters of the beds for the tuberculous were local, state, or federal, the rest being private.(22)

In 1917 the U.S. Department of Agriculture instituted a national program for the eradication of tuberculosis among cattle. Bovine tuberculosis was a source of economic loss to the cattle industry and, it was well established by this time, a health hazard for people, especially children. The federal-state program involved the tuberculin testing of cattle, the slaughter of infected animals, indemnification for their owners, regulation of the movement of cattle, and the accrediting of areas where the infection rate was reduced to less than 0.5 percent. The whole country became an accredited area in 1940 when the overall rate of infection was 0.46 percent. Bovine tuberculosis was at all times less common in the United States than Britain, and its complete eradication more nearly achieved: the proportion of infected cattle in 1949 was still 21.3 percent in England, but only 5.4 percent in Wales. In the United States, only 4.9 percent of tested cattle reacted to tuberculin in 1918, the first full year of the federal-state program, and by 1949 that figure had dropped to 0.19.(23)

Notwithstanding the success of state intervention in eradicating bovine tuberculosis, the federal role was much more limited than that of the central government in Britain, and in general voluntary efforts played a more important role in the country's control of tuberculosis. The National Tuberculosis Association (NTA) at first distrusted official public health bodies as being too "political," having no personnel standards, and tending to undermine voluntary efforts.(24) State, and especially municipal, boards of health had earned poor reputations in the nineteenth century as ineffective and corrupt bodies of unqualified political appointees.(25) They were among the less salubrious manifestations of the spoils system.*

Gradually and unevenly, the NTA and other voluntary associations came to support an extension of the state's role in controlling tuberculosis, through providing beds and clinics, case finding, and other activities. During and after World War I there were moves to bring about a tuberculosis division in the U.S. Public Health Service, but the Kent Bill of 1917, which would have provided for this, failed to pass despite NTA support, as did similar bills in the following legislative session. Increasingly the NTA became a force for greater involvement and action by the state, especially at the federal level. The financial scale of the problem pushed them in this direction, as did the situation of migrant consumptives, who failed to meet the residency requirements for state and local provision. This problem would increase greatly in the 1930s and featured prominently in demands for more extensive federal action.(26)

Lacking the impetus of national health insurance, the role of the American central government was largely confined to the bovine tuberculosis program, and to provision for the armed forces and veterans. World War I was an important stimulus. Even before

---

*The discussions surrounding the establishment of a tuberculosis division within the Ohio State Board of Health reveal the ambivalence of the voluntary antituberculosis movement toward state intervention. According to the historian of the NTA, Richard Shryock, the Ohio Tuberculosis Association in 1912 persuaded the state legislature to set up a special division within the state health board. But Robert G. Paterson, a member of the Ohio association and at the time of writing these comments secretary of the NTA's Committee on Archives, noted that:

Leaders of the National Tuberculosis Association were fearful of such a proposal on three grounds. It was feared first, that such a step would throw the tuberculosis movement into politics; second, that professional personnel requirements in state Boards of Health were nonexistent, or on such a low plane that little or no help would accrue to the movement; and third, that the creation of such an official agency would constitute a threat to private tuberculosis control activities. (Paterson, "Official Tuberculosis Control," p. 339; Shryock, National Tuberculosis Association, p. 125.)

American entry into the war, alarming, and not always accurate, reports of widespread tuberculosis in the French army prompted cooperation between the NTA and the government with regard to the screening of draftees, treatment for infected rejects (whose data were forwarded to the Red Cross), and preventive and educational measures. The government took responsibility for infected soldiers and veterans and began, in 1919, an extensive hospital-building program to provide residential treatment for veterans. The program was expensive and controversial. Of nearly 11,000 beds available by 1923, 2,500 were vacant, mainly due to the remote location of the Veterans Bureau hospitals. For the same reason, some 40 percent of patients discharged themselves against medical advice. The NTA had argued in vain for using the federal dollars to expand existing local institutions, instead of building large federal hospitals far from veterans' homes and families.(27)

Many developments in the 1930s seemed to point in the direction of a more comprehensive attack on tuberculosis, coordinated and in large part funded by the federal government. The feasibility and potential of such a program seemed greater as incidence of the disease continued to decline, and developments in medical treatment and research (such as the work of Selman Waksman and René Dubos on soil microbiology and antibiotics) made tuberculosis appear more than ever a conquerable disease rather than an inevitable part of the human condition. Social and epidemiological aspects of the disease were studied intensively, and more exact knowledge of mortality and morbidity was attained.(28) The importance, and possibility, of early diagnosis and treatment became more clearly apparent. Technological developments in X-ray photography made mass screening feasible, and extended the possibilities of case finding beyond examinations of contacts.(29)

The Depression itself seemed to increase the probability of a larger federal role in tuberculosis control, as it did in other areas. State and local governments lost much of their tax base, and voluntary organizations found it harder to raise money. NTA finances suffered: between 1932 and 1938 there was a serious decline in income from the association's principal funding source, the sale of Christmas seals.(30) Much of the resistance to federal intervention in health and welfare gave way before the weight of the crisis. Roosevelt's New Deal produced a range of temporary and permanent federal or federal-state programs, most importantly those of the 1935 Social Security Act.

The Depression also produced an increase in the migrant population, including the tuberculous who did not meet the residency requirements of local tuberculosis institutions, but who spread infection and needed treatment. This problem fueled demands for federal aid.(31) The Committee on the Costs of Medical Care, which carried out a very extensive investigation between 1927 and 1932, and produced 27 field studies (and 28 reports), cast new light on the general problem of unmet medical need. This and other efforts by researchers and reformers gave new hope that some form of government health insurance would be forthcoming, perhaps as part of the Social Security Act. The movement of many social workers and reformers with direct experience of tuberculosis work into federal government service also offered hope of national action. Most important in this respect was the appointment as head of the Federal Emergency Relief Administration of Harry Hopkins, who had been executive officer of the New York City Tuberculosis and Health Association (an outgrowth of the earlier committee of the COS) and, in 1929, president of the National Conference of Tuberculosis Secretaries.(32)

These hopes did not go wholly unrealized. Insofar as the New Deal's income maintenance programs succeeded in maintaining income, they helped the tuberculous, their families, and those who might otherwise have succumbed. The same is true of the food and nutrition programs discussed in the preceding chapter. Child health and home nursing activities were undertaken as disease prevention measures by the FERA and Civil Works Administration. Provision of free medical care to those on relief removed some of the financial barrier to early diagnosis and treatment. The U.S. Public Health Service began epidemiological studies in 1936 to explore the reasons for the very great geographical, age, sex, and race variation in tuberculosis mortality, a fact that came to general awareness as the disease declined.(33)

But all this amounted to much less than a comprehensive federal antituberculosis program. State and local health departments, while accounting for most of the country's tuberculosis beds, often had very weak and poorly funded control and prevention programs. Most states had no full-time director or tuberculosis control officers. State and local health departments lacked funds for case finding and hospitalization of the seriously ill.(34) There was still a shortage and maldistribution of beds in 1940, twelve states not having reached the modest goal of ensuring as many beds as there were annual deaths from the disease.(35) Beds were not always entirely free and, where they were, sometimes carried the stigma of pauperism. The main direct federal effort was for veterans. While many New Deal programs impinged on tuberculosis control, little was done specifically for the tuberculous. There was a growing awareness of the special, additional income needs of sufferers and their families, and also of the importance of vocational rehabilitation, but little concerted government action.(36) For the most part, then, the "promise" of the thirties in regard to the nationalization and centralization of tuberculosis control was not fulfilled. Tuberculosis remained a terrible drain on the nation's productive manpower, however, and though that was not in itself a problem in a period of mass unemployment, World War II would make it a compelling reason for state intervention.

WORLD WAR II

War made of tuberculosis an urgent problem for the state. Past experience taught that wars tended to result in increased infection and mortality, the more so as they increasingly disrupted normal life. People were more exposed to infection, through close interaction in the armed forces, air raid shelters, refugee camps and temporary facilities for the homeless, in industrial plants, and so forth. Nutrition might be undermined by the interruption of food supplies. While troops suffered the stress, anxiety, and often exhaustion of war, workers would work long hours in hastily converted factories with inadequate standards of hygiene. Such factors were certainly held responsible for the increase in tuberculosis in World War I in Britain and other combatant countries.

If the social conditions of war were likely to exacerbate the problem of tuberculosis, the state's dependence on healthy, fit workers and soldiers in a situation of acute labor shortage made tuberculosis a problem for the state. It did not, especially at first, seem the most pressing health problem, however. Fearing heavy civilian bombing and increased demand for hospital beds for both the military and civilian wounded, the British government adopted a policy of diverting resources from the tuberculosis service to more urgent needs.

Tuberculosis officers became air raid wardens, sanatoria became war hospitals, patients went home, care committee members took on other tasks, nursing and medical staff joined the armed forces. Local authorities surpassed the Ministry of Health's intentions in turning patients out of their beds. Every such patient (8,000, some highly infectious, were discharged from sanatoria, while there were 70,000 sputum positive cases on the dispensary registers, 10,000 of them in London)(37) was a radiating center of infection. Or, as the British Medical Journal put it in a wartime metaphor, "Every tuberculous person turned forth is like a bomb thrown among the public."(38)

As concern mounted at this situation, and local reports began to show a rising mortality from tuberculosis, official efforts were made to restore the functioning of the tuberculosis service and to return sanatorium beds for use by the tuberculous. These efforts, including the release of 6,000 beds, were beginning to take effect by the spring of 1940, when the war itself intervened in the form of the long expected civilian bombing. As hospital beds were again emptied of the tuberculous, and now filled with casualites and the chronic sick from danger areas, many highly infectious tuberculosis patients joined their neighbors in crowded public air raid shelters, including the London Underground.(39)

War did not disrupt American tuberculosis services so greatly, but there was official concern about its impact on efforts to control the disease. By the time of American entry into the war, it was evident that tuberculosis mortality had risen substantially in England and Wales (6 percent in the first year of the war, and 10 percent in the second), still more in Scotland, and had reached epidemic proportions in France.(40) Some of the most important factors in the British increase did not, as experts in the United States pointed out, apply to the American situation. Sanatoria did not evacuate their patients and distribute them among the general public, while bovine tuberculosis, the source of much of the mortality from nonpulmonary tuberculosis among children, was more nearly eradicated in the United States.(41) Nevertheless, several other factors seemed to pose a threat to tuberculosis control. The drain of civilian doctors and nurses to the military extended to sanatoria and other tuberculosis facilities, making it still more difficult to ensure that patients in need of residential treatment could receive it promptly. It also produced fears that civilian health in general would suffer, and, with it, resistance to tubercular infection. Residence qualifications became more than ever an obstacle to the treatment of an increasingly mobile population. The war-boom towns, with poor, overcrowded living conditions and long hours of work, provided a setting conducive to the spread of tuberculosis while the labor shortage drew infected workers into the factories.(42)

In both countries, the state responded to the challenge of tuberculosis in wartime with new official bodies and activities, providing a more comprehensive control program coordinated at the national level of government. In 1939, the British minister of health set up a Standing Advisory Committee on Tuberculosis, after meeting with tuberculosis workers from various official and voluntary bodies, including the National Association for the Prevention of Tuberculosis, the Joint Tuberculosis Council, and the Tuberculosis Association. The committee, which spawned two important subcommittees, on mass radiography and tuberculin testing, reported to the minister on tuberculosis services in war conditions. One of its earliest actions was to press for the release of forcibly evacuated sanatorium beds.(43)

At the Ministry of Health's request, the Medical Research Council set up a Committee on Tuberculosis in War-Time. This was a response to the early indications of increased incidence and mortality, and the committee was charged "to assist in promoting an investigation of the extent and causes of the wartime increase in the incidence of tuberculosis, particularly among young women, and also to advise the Council regarding possible preventive measures."(44) The committee documented the increase, but found that all age groups were affected, that, unlike World War I, it was older males rather than young women who suffered the largest increase, that the increase included nonpulmonary as well as pulmonary tuberculosis, especially in the form of childhood mortality from meningitis. Its recommendations included the use of mass miniature radiography, particularly in the armed services, the war industries, and certain other occupations; examination of contacts, including all home contacts; special financial provision for the tuberculous; additional residential facilities and the recruitment of more nursing and domestic staff; pasteurization of milk; improvements in general working conditions; and rehabilitation, seen as an essential part of treatment.(45) The government attempted to carry out most of these recommendations: Its actions are discussed later in this chapter.

Soon after American entry into the war the National Tuberculosis Association appointed a War Emergency Committee, and the Surgeon General, Thomas Parran, established an office of tuberculosis control in the U.S. Public Health Service. A subcommittee on tuberculosis within the medical division of the National Research Council advised the military. There was considerable overlap of membership between these committees: Dr. Herman E. Hilleboe, a member of the NTA's War Emergency Committee (WEC), became head of the Public Health Service's office of tuberculosis control, while Dr. Esmond R. Long, former president of the NTA and also a member of its WEC, was made chief consultant on tuberculosis in the office of the surgeon general of the army. NTA leaders thus became not simply advisers to the government, but part of the state apparatus at national executive level. As Shryock notes:

> Through such appointments the Association in effect infiltrated strategic federal centers concerned with tuberculosis control. It therefore may be said to have guided federal policy from within, rather than as an outside agency as during World War I.(46)

The work of the office of tuberculosis control in the U.S. Public Health Service had the status of a war emergency program. It concentrated on the mass screening of war workers, on developing a referral system whereby active cases detected by industrial or military screening might be referred to state and local health departments, and on improving X-ray technology.(47) Its work, combined with the propaganda efforts of the NTA, whetted the long unrequited appetite for permanent federal leadership of and responsibility for tuberculosis control. In July 1944 the Public Health Service Act (PL 78-410) at last granted what had been denied in 1917, congressional authorization for the establishment of a federal tuberculosis control program. The Public Health Service, through its Tuberculosis Control Division, became responsible for administering grants-in-aid to state health departments and for conducting demonstrations and research in tuberculosis.(48) Thenceforth the federal government was to play a leading role in coordinating and funding tuberculosis control, emphasizing especially case finding, prevention, and long-term research.

Screening

War involved in both countries the mobilization of all available human resources. Millions were drafted into the armed services, while other millions became workers in the war industries. Case finding in these circumstances took on a change of emphasis and a new importance. It became a matter of protecting the valuable manpower, on which the state depended, from debilitation. Tuberculosis appeared as a destructive force capable of immense damage to the war effort, at home and abroad. It operated like the much talked about "fifth column." Its agents were everywhere, and they might be young or old, male or female. A telltale cough might give one away, but often there was no obvious way to distinguish them from the fit and healthy beside whom they worked and fought. They had to be detected before the danger spread.

In both countries, but especially in Britain, the need to screen the nation's manpower had far-reaching implications. It gave a strong stimulus to the application and refinement of the new X-ray technology, which now made it possible, by taking and examining a photograph, to detect disease at a much earlier stage than had been possible in World War I with even the most thorough physical examination. X-rays could reveal disease when the subject was not aware of any symptoms. Screening for war would thus greatly develop case finding in peace, and give it a central place in tuberculosis control.

Unlike enemy agents, however, those detected with tuberculosis could not, for obvious reasons, be shot, imprisoned, or recruited as double agents. The more new active cases the screening of military conscripts and industrial workers brought to light, the more it increased the pressure for adequate treatment and rehabilitation facilities, as well as for financial provision that would maintain income without the necessity of work. Simply discovering thousands of previously undetected tuberculous people posed the question of what the state was going to do about them.

Highest priority was given, in both countries, to screening those drafted for or already in military service. Routine X-ray screening of recruits did not become fully established until 1943, the year in which mass radiography of civilian populations developed. Its importance for the military is indicated by the drop in the tuberculosis admission rate in the U.S. army hospitals, from 3.0 per thousand per year in December 1941, before systematic X-ray screening, to 0.8 percent by 1944 (less than one-tenth of the rate during World War I).(49) Military and industrial screening together, in the United States, led to the discovery of about 140,000 previously undiagnosed cases of tuberculosis by early 1944, about half of which were active.(50) Mass X-ray screening developed less rapidly in Britain, perhaps because of the expense and difficulties involved in supplying and equipping mass miniature radiography units.

By the end of 1945, about 797,000 persons had undergone X-ray examination. Of these, 2,915 (3.7 per thousand) were diagnosed as having previously unsuspected active pulmonary tuberculosis, and another 15,655 as cases of quiescent or inactive tuberculosis.(51)

American servicemen who were diagnosed as tuberculous became the responsibility of the armed services, and later of the Veterans Administration. They were treated in military and veterans' hospitals. Draftees who were rejected because of tuberculosis diagnosed at induction centers received the help of medical social workers and others in finding treatment from state and local sources. New cases uncovered by draft examinations and industrial surveys were reported to state health departments. One result of the mass screening effort was to widen the gap between case finding and follow-up facilities. The states and localities were ill equipped to handle 140,000 new cases. Only about half the states had full-time medical tuberculosis officers and essential clinic facilities.(52) Another result was that the military and the Veterans Administration were saved the ongoing expense of caring for thousands of tuberculous draftees, who were screened out by preinduction medical examination.(53)

In Britain tuberculous members of the armed services were removed as quickly as possible from military hospitals. The Ministry of Health developed, in 1941, a central allocation scheme, which, by the end of the war, had organized the transfer of about 10,000 service cases to civilian treatment facilities within reasonable reach of the patients' homes.(54) Here too, lack of beds, and especially their unavailability due to staffing shortages, meant that patients needing residential treatment could not always receive it promptly.

Even where adequate facilities and treatment were available, patients in both countries tended to discharge themselves against medical advice. Several factors contributed to this problem, including, in the United States, the location of many treatment facilities at considerable distances from patients' homes and families. Of great importance was the need of tuberculous bread-winners to meet their own and their families' financial needs. Keeping them out of the work force in a period of acute labor shortage was a difficult matter. American industry achieved it, in part, by widely making X-ray screening a condition of employment, and then refusing to hire the tuberculous. Case finding became, in that context, a method of marking individuals with a stigma. In Britain, one attempt to deal with this problem was the development, as a war emergency measure, of an income maintenance program to make special financial provision for the tuberculous cases who might otherwise be in the work force. It was a solution full of problems, paradoxes, and contradictions.

The Tuberculosis Allowances Scheme

In applying mass radiography to the civilian population, the British government hoped both to bring about the removal from the work force of those with infectious tuberculosis and to ensure their speedy return to work after successful treatment. X-rays made it possible to detect and treat the disease at an earlier stage than had previously been possible, and so held out the promise of reducing the spread of infection to others while improving the prognosis for the infected individual. The problem was to persuade workers who felt few or no symptoms of disease to leave work and undergo prolonged treatment. In seeking to gain acceptance of its mass radiography campaign, the government insisted on the confidentiality of the results, and rejected compulsion either to undergo X-ray examination or to give up work if it revealed active tuberculosis.

In its 1942 report, the Medical Research Council's Committee on Tuberculosis in War-Time had emphasized the special character of the disease.(55) It particularly affected the productive part of the population, and usually lasted for more than six months. But after six months the sickness benefit from national health insurance dropped from 18 shillings to 10 shillings and 6 pence. Tuberculosis tended to reduce the standard of living of patient and family, yet required a relatively high standard of living, with nutritious food, adequate housing conditions, and so forth, for successful treatment and to increase the family's resistance. Freedom from economic worries was, in the committee's view, important for successful treatment and for the prevention of a relapse. For these reasons, it recommended that special financial provision, greater than that allowed for by national health insurance, be made for the tuberculous and their families.

In May 1943, the Ministry of Health announced its tuberculosis allowances scheme. A wartime measure "which did not purport to be comprehensive," it was "framed primarily to assist patients, who undertake early treatment instead of continuing to work at the risk of breakdown, to meet their necessary financial commitments during a limited period of treatment."(56) The beneficiary was required to follow the treatment that was prescribed, and to have the "prospect of ultimate restoration to full working capacity."(57) The scheme provided for payments of nearly two pounds per week, with additional amounts for dependents, without a means test. Actual rent and property taxes up to 15 shillings per week, and fuel allowance in winter were also paid, as well as certain discretionary allowances and special payments. The program was universal insofar as the standard allowance did not involve a means test and so was not confined to the poor. It was also clearly differentiated from public assistance of the poor law variety by being defined as an integral part of treatment. Beneficiaries received their payments from the local tuberculosis dispensary.

As Ferguson and Fitzgerald show in their detailed account of the scheme, it was the outcome of an understanding reached between the Treasury and the Ministry of Health.(58) The Treasury was concerned that the program might set a precedent for all the disabled, that it breached the means test principle, and that it might establish a higher rate of benefits than would be available under the comprehensive, universal social insurance system that was being introduced piecemeal from 1945 on, and had been agreed in principle by 1943. The Ministry of Health adopted a stretegy of "anticipatory surrender," to use Arnold Kaufman's term.(59) They anticipated Treasury objections to extending the coverage and improving the level of payments under the program, and did not push for such reforms.

Conditions of war had made the Treasury, with other sections of the government, recognize the special character of tuberculosis. The allowances scheme was justified, but also limited, by the economic needs of war production. Its aim was to encourage workers with active tuberculosis to leave their jobs and undergo treatment, both to remove infection from the work place and to provide for early treatment and a return to the labor force of badly needed workers. The scheme was thus explicitly a manpower program, and the criteria of eligibility were that the disease be infectious (i.e. pulmonary) and curable. Those with chronic pulmonary tuberculosis were excluded as being beyond restoration to the work force, even though they might be highly infectious and forced by economic necessity to return to or remain at work. Nonpulmonary cases, on the other hand, were excluded, along with other types of disability, because they were not infectious, even though they might be recoverable for the labor force. By the application of both these criteria together, infectiousness and "curability," the large majority of the tuberculous were excluded from the scheme.

The demands of economic efficiency alone might seem to have indicated the inclusion of chronic cases of pulmonary tuberculosis, because of the danger of infection they represented. Ministry of Health officials dismissed this arguement as not being feasible: it would involve "transferring the cost of maintenance from Public Assistance to Public Health," which was "outside the scope of a war service grant," and would also be too costly to be acceptable to the Treasury."(60)

Not fully consistent even in strictly economic or efficiency terms, the scheme involved serious problems of legitimation. The task of distinguishing the chronics from those who stood a reasonable chance of recovery fell to the local tuberculosis officers. To be judged chronic, and hence ineligible for allowance, was in effect to be told that one would die of the disease, and that the government did not consider one worth investing in.

In dealing with an illness where morale was an important factor, physicians felt they were being asked to pass a death sentence on their patients. Welcomed at first as a recognition of the importance of adequate living standards of the whole family for the treatment and prevention of tuberculosis, and as a universal program without the taint of the poor law, the allowances scheme roused great bitterness once its limitations were realized. In providing payments only for those who might recover and rejoin the work force – in being so strictly an investment in labor power – it appeared callous and cruel, not only to patients and their families, but also to those involved in administering the program.

Those with active pulmonary tuberculosis at an early stage where recovery seemed likely were clearly a minority of those known to be tuberculous. But the rates at which patients were judged eligible for the scheme varied greatly. Some local authorities used funds from other sources to blanket in most tuberculous patients. Although the Ministry of Health would not support extension of coverage, it turned a blind eye to these local practices, even after ascertaining that they were illegal.

The government intended the level of benefits to be higher than could be obtained from national health insurance or public assistance. They based their thinking on recognition of the special needs of the tuberculous and their families, and more particularly on what might be called the principle of more eligibility. That is, they hoped to make not working more attractive to the tuberculous than going to work. They would do this by educating those with active but early tuberculosis about the long-term advantages of early treatment as opposed to continuing at work until forced by illness to undergo lengthier treatment with a poorer prognosis; and by making the cessation of work more immediately appealing through a relatively high level of benefits.

In practice, however, the level of the tuberculosis allowance was no higher than public assistance in some areas, though, not being subject to a means test, it benefitted most those who were ineligible for poor law payments. The allowances were not substantially altered until 1947, despite inflation. After public assistance scales were revised in December 1943, the child of an unemployed worker received a higher benefit than the child of a tuberculous patient, an anomaly that was not removed until December 1946. Ferguson and Fitzgerald explain this failure to establish and maintain levels of benefit in line with the principles of the scheme by pointing to the emerging system of social security. "In 1943," they point out, "the Government had accepted the general principles of the Beveridge Report – that is, the abolition of the Poor Law and the replacement of the old assessment of needs and the patchwork of unequal benefits by a unified system of payments made as of right."(61) When that system was fully established, all tuberculous patients, whatever the type or severity of their disease, would receive a national minimum sickness benefit, allowances for their children, full treatment under the national health service, and supplementary payments if necessary from the projected National Assistance Board. From July 1948, payments to those who suffered loss of income in order to undergo treatment for pulmonary tuberculosis were taken over by the National Assistance Board, and the allowances scheme came to an end.(62)

In the meantime, however, civil servants were concerned not to undermine the unity of the postwar social insurance system, which would make a minimum payment to all, without a means test, in the event of sickness or disability. The Ministry of Health became increasingly aware of the anomalies and inadequacy of the tuberculosis allowances scheme, but would not, according to Ferguson and Fitzgerald, propose improvement to the Treasury, "which was reported to be very sensitive to any suggestion that tuberculosis rates might exceed corresponding rates under the postwar social insurance schemes."(63)

In other related areas of social policy, such as nutrition or rehabilitation, war stimulated a substantial increase in the extent and generosity of social provision. By contrast, the tuberculosis allowances scheme was discriminatory and meager. On the one hand it was so directly and immediately tied to the function of ensuring the adequacy of the labor supply that it appeared callous and inhumane, almost like part of a Nazi eugenics program. On the other hand, the developing unified system of social security, itself in part a response to the stimulus of war, became the reason for keeping the allowances at a level that was wholly inadequate in terms of the scheme's purpose.

The Ministry of Health recognized that the program was anomalous, contradictory, and inadequate. It felt powerless, however, to come up with a rational revision of the scheme that had any chance of being accepted. It could not resolve the conflicting claims of fiscal economy, manpower, and legitimation, or the conflicts within the tuberculosis officer "between official obligation and professional duty to the patient."(64) In response to the latter problem, it simply explained that it was aware of the dilemma, "but the Minister, if given money by Parliament for war services, could not spend it in ways that could not possibly be regarded as war service."(65) Ministry officials defended the scheme as the best that could be done at the time. It was "part of the price of doing something, at least, for the tuberculous immediately, rather than doing nothing at all until something better could be done when the war was over."(66)

Whether doing nothing was the only alternative is doubtful, but it is clear that the price of "doing something," or rather this particular thing, was, in terms of legitimation and rationality, a high one. Nevertheless, the unfortunate scheme shows the strength of the impulse to do something, anything, to relieve the manpower situation, and at the same time, the difficulties that were likely to arise if such social policy interventions were too strictly limited by manpower considerations alone.

Tuberculosis and War

War did not produce the dramatic increases in tuberculosis rates, in Britain or the United States, that many had feared. In Britain, the pattern of increase was alarmingly similar, from 1939 to 1941, to what it had been in 1914 to 1916. "But whereas in 1917 mortality showed a fresh rise which was further considerably increased in 1918, the years 1942 and 1943 showed a smart fall to the prewar level. The 1944 figures show a continuance of the fall to a new record low level."(67) The downward trend continued in 1945 and accelerated in subsequent years. In the United States, the downward trend of the twenties and thirties continued through the war years, despite a rise in some industrial states like Massachusetts. In the postwar years, major advances in chemotherapy (the use of streptomycin beginning in the war, combined with other drugs, especially, from the early fifties, isoniazid), the expansion and refinement of public health control measures, and the doubling of real incomes in 20 years, all combined to produce a dramatic drop in tuberculosis rates in both countries.(68) Of these factors the last, with its concomitant improvement in general levels of housing and nutrition, was probably the most important.(69)

As we have seen, the war generated or strengthened many tendencies favorable to the spread of tuberculosis, especially in Britain. But there were also countertendencies. Real incomes, employment opportunities, even nutrition, improved, and important advances in these respects were made by those sections of the population most prone to tuberculosis.

Furthermore, the war, in making tuberculosis a problem for the state, elicited strong governmental intervention. In both countries the process of centralizing tuberculosis control at the national level of government was greatly advanced, a process that continued after the war, with the National Health Service in Britain and the expanded federal role in financing hospital construction and medical research and training in the United States.(70)

The need to screen the nation's manpower for military and industrial purposes exposed gaps and problems in treatment facilities, as well as saving the Veterans Administration a great deal of money. Screening on such a scale and with such effect was made possible by, but it also stimulated, technological advances in radiography. The British government, while unable to reduce the prevalence of bovine tuberculosis to a level close to American rates before federal intervention in 1917, went far toward eliminating the infection of the human population through milk. It published two white papers dealing with milk policy, in 1942 and 1943 set up a National Milk Testing and Advisory Scheme, and issued Defence Regulation 55G, requiring in effect that all milk be tuberculin-tested, accredited (from one infection-free herd), pasteurized, or sterilized.(71)

War certainly stimulated state involvement in the rehabilitation and employment of the disabled, including the tuberculous. Tuberculosis workers were aware of the importance of rehabilitation in the 1930s, but as Shryock puts it, "the public was not inclined to worry much about opportunities for the handicapped when there were millions of healthy persons unemployed."(72) Like shale oil or a difficult mine, however, the disabled of all kinds became worth exploiting when the resource, in this case labor power, was expensive and in short supply.(73) The war itself swelled the ranks of the disabled with new recruits from the battlefields and war plants, reinforcing economic considerations with political obligation.

Both governments subsidized and assisted the rehabilitation of disabled people during the war to a much greater extent than ever before. New programs and legislation, including the Vocational Rehabilitation Act of 1943 in the United States and the Disabled Persons Act of 1944 in Britain, extended the state's role in rehabilitating the tuberculous, who had often been excluded from earlier programs.(74) There were special problems in tuberculosis rehabilitation, such as the danger of relapse and the consequent spreading of infection. Little progress was made during the war itself, but under the pressure of manpower needs and the political obligation to those disabled by war, a new level of government responsibility was established, for the disabled in general and incidentally for the tuberculous. The Disabled Persons Act was especially important for state-capital relations in this area: it empowered the state to force employers to take a prescribed quota of rehabilitated workers.(75)

In an appendix to their book, The White Plague, René and Jean Dubos show how World War II interrupted the trend of declining tuberculosis mortality in Britain for almost ten years.(76) But if we examine, as we have here, the trend of increasing state involvement in tuberculosis control, we find a great acceleration during, and largely because of, the war. War did not, in this case, enhance the health of the people, though it did not harm it as much as expected. But it did strengthen the role of the state. In the United States, as we saw, the war had little overall effect on declining tuberculosis rates, although the trend was reversed in some areas. Whatever its effect on the people's health, however, war proved in both countries to be "the health of the state."(77)

NOTES

(1)   Sheila Ferguson and Hilde Fitzgerald, Studies in the Social Services, p. 261.

(2)   "Yet the Captain of all these men of death that came against him to take him away, was the Consumption, for 'twas that brought him down to the grave." John Bunyan, The Life and Death of Mr. Badman (1680), London: Oxford University Press, 1929, p. 239.

(3) Ferguson and Fitzgerald, Studies, pp. 251-52; PEP (Political and Economic Planning), Report on British Health Service, p. 282-85; René and Jean Dubos, The White Plague, pp. 186, 199-207, passim; René Dubos, Mirage of Health, pp. 191-94; Thomas McKeown, Medicine in Modern Society, pp. 43-50; idem, The Role of Medicine, pp. 61, 65, 92-96.

(4) W. M. Frazer, History of English Public Health, p. 315.

(5) Ibid., p. 319.

(6) See Frank Honigsbaum, Struggle for Ministry of Health, p. 12.

(7) Honigsbaum, Struggle for Ministry of Health, p. 62.

(8) PEP, British Health Services, pp. 285-86; Frazer, English Public Health, p. 318.

(9) Frazer, English Public Health, p. 426; PEP, British Health Services, p. 286.

(10) PEP, British Health Services, pp. 282-85.

(11) Medical Research Council, Report of the Committee on Tuberculosis in War-Time, 1942, p. 5a

(12) PEP, British Health Services, p. 282.

(13) R. and J. Dubos, White Plague, p. 171.

(14) PEP, British Health Services, p. 288.

(15) Ibid.

(16) Sir Arthur MacNalty, ed., Civilian Health and Medical Services, p. 101.

(17) John Boyd Orr and J. L. Gilks, "The Physique and Health of Two African Tribes," Medical Research Council, Special Report, Series No. 155, London, 1931. See also J. B. McDougall, Tuberculosis, p. 359.

(18) Dubos, White Plague, pp. 185-86; Anthony M. Lowell, Tuberculosis, pp. 15-16; E.T. Blomquist, "Prospect of Tuberculosis Eradication," Public Health Reports 78 (1963): 507-09; Godias J. Drolet, "Epidemiology of Tuberculosis."

(19) Daniel Fox, "Social Policy and City Politics," pp. 169-95; Walter I. Trattner, From Poor Law to Welfare State, pp. 124-25.

(20) Trattner, From Poor Law to Welfare State, p. 125. For the history of the National Tuberculosis Association, see Richard Harrison Shryock, National Tuberculosis Association 1904-1954.

(21) "An Index to State Tuberculosis Laws," Public Health Reports 38 (1923): 1191-1200.

(22) Philip P. Jacobs, "72,000 Beds for Tuberculosis Treatment," American City 39 (1928): 98. Cf. Lowell, Tuberculosis, p. 32.

(23) Dubos, White Plague, pp. 109-10, 259-60 n. 6; Lowell, Tuberculosis; pp. 20-21; MacNalty, Civilian Health, p. 101; J. Arthur Myers, Man's Greatest Victory; John Francis, Bovine Tuberculosis; James A. Tobey, National Government and Public Health, p. 200.

(24) Robert G. Paterson, "Evolution of Official Tuberculosis Control," p. 339.

(25) Trattner, From Poor Law, p. 118. Trattner notes that six of seven members of Cincinnati's board of health were saloon-keepers.

(26) Paterson, "Official Tuberculosis Control," p. 340.
(27) Shryock, National Tuberculosis Association, pp. 175-81.
(28) Ibid., pp. 251-55.
(29) Ibid., p. 237.
(30) Ibid., p. 227.
(31) Paterson, "Official Tuberculosis Control," p. 340.
(32) Shryock, National Tuberculosis Association, p. 227.
(33) L.L. Lumsden and W.P. Dearing, "Epidemiological Studies of Tuberculosis," pp. 219-28.
(34) Shryock, National Tuberculosis Association, pp. 233, 263; Harry S. Mustard, Government in Public Health, pp. 151-55.
(35) Ibid., p. 154.
(36) See, for example, W.H. Frost, "How Much Control of Tuberculosis?" American Journal of Public Health 27 (1937): 759-66; A. Frances Beery, "An Experiment in Treatment of Tuberculosis Patients," Social Forces 16 (1938): 523-27; Alice L. Moore, "Health So Hardly Won," Survey Midmonthly 75 (1939): 43-44.
(37) Ferguson and Fitzgerald, Studies, pp. 254-55.
(38) Quoted by Ferguson and Fitzgerald, ibid., p. 254.
(39) Ferguson and Fitzgerald, Studies, p. 225.
(40) Percy Stocks, "Vital Statistics of the Second Year of the War," Lancet 242 (1942), p. 190; idem, "Tuberculosis Deaths and the War," British Medical Journal 26 (1943), pp. 750-51; Thomas Parran, "Outlook for Tuberculosis Control in the Civilian Population," Transactions, New York, NTA, 1944, p. 144.
(41) Shryock, National Tuberculosis Association, pp. 261-62.
(42) Ibid., p. 262; Paterson, "Official Tuberculosis Control," p. 340.
(43) MacNalty, Civilian Health, p. 93; Ferguson and Fitzgerald, Studies, p. 225.
(44) U.K. Medical Research Council, Report of Committee on Tuberculosis in War-Time, p. ii.
(45) U.K. Medical Research Council, Tuberculosis in War-Time, pp. 29-30.
(46) Shryock, National Tuberculosis Association, p. 260.
(47) Henry D. Chadwick and Alton S. Pope, Modern Attack on Tuberculosis, p. 90.
(48) Lowell, Tuberculosis, pp. 13-14.
(49) Esmond R. Long, "Tuberculosis and the War," pp. 178-79.
(50) Ibid., p. 177.
(51) MacNalty, Civilian Health, pp. 106-7; Ministry of Health, Report of the Ministry of Health for the Year Ended 31st March 1946 (Cnd 7119), London: HMSO 1946.
(52) Shryock, National Tuberculosis Association, p. 263.
(53) Saul Solomon, Tuberculosis, pp. 257-58.
(54) U.K. Ministry of Health, On the State of Public Health, pp. 62-63.
(55) U.K. Medical Research Council, Tuberculosis in War-Time, pp. 20-21.
(56) U.K. Ministry of Health, On the State of Public Health, p. 65.
(57) Ibid.
(58) Ferguson and Fitzgerald, Studies, pp. 258-73.

(59) Arnold S. Kaufman, The Radical Liberal, pp. 30-32.

(60) Ferguson and Fitzgerald, Studies, p. 281, n. 2.

(61) Ibid., p. 273.

(62) Ibid., p. 275, n. 5.

(63) Ibid., p. 273.

(64) U.K. Ministry of Health, On the State of Public Health, p. 65.

(65) Ibid.

(66) Ibid.

(67) Ibid., p. 59. Cf. MacNalty, Civilian Health, pp. 90-91.

(68) Lowell, Tuberculosis, pp. 45-93, 99-100.

(69) But Cf. McKeown, Role of Medicine, pp. 95-96, who emphasizes the medicine's postwar contribution to increasing the decline of mortality rates.

(70) Cf. Louis S. Reed and Edward T. Blomquist, "Tuberculosis Facilities and Planning Under the Hospital Survey and Construction Act," Public Health Reports 65 (1950): 146-54.

(71) MacNalty, Civilian Health, pp. 101-2.

(72) Shryock, National Tuberculosis Association, p. 247.

(73) Cf. Angus Calder, People's War, p. 447.

(74) See Ferguson and Fitzgerald, Studies, pp. 276-79; Shryock, National Tuberculosis Association, pp. 248-49, 263; Herman E. Hilleboe and Norvin C. Kiefer, "Rehabilitation and Aftercare," pp. 285-94.

(75) Richard M. Titmuss, Problems of Social Policy, pp. 476-80; H.M.D. Parker, Manpower, pp. 267-70.

(76) Dubos, White Plague, Appendix C.

(77) Randolph Bourne, War and the Intellectuals, p. 71.

7

REFORMING MORALS AND
MAKING FORNICATION SAFE:
VENEREAL DISEASE CONTROL

There are many similarities between venereal disease and tuber-culosis, seen as health problems confronting the state.* Both tend to increase in wartime, and both had increased in World War I. Both attacked men and women in their productive years and were major drains on manpower.

In Britain and the United States the state responded to the venereal disease problem in ways similar to those adopted for tuberculosis control. An international voluntary health movement, which spawned the National Council for Combating Venereal Diseases (1915) in Britain and the American Social Hygiene Association (1914) in the United States, pressed for recognition of the problem and for government action. The possibility of controlling venereal disease presented itself with the development in 1910 of an apparently effective, if protracted and dangerous, treatment for syphilis, called salvarsan (later arsphenamine).† The wartime epidemic in the armed forces of all combatant countries (which caused a loss of some 7 million man days in the U.S. Army alone) demonstrated the necessity of controlling venereal disease.

A Royal Commission on Venereal Diseases was appointed in Britain in 1913. It reported in 1916, by which time war had made the

---

*For the sake of simplicity, I use "venereal diseases" to mean syphilis and gonorrhea, although there are several other, much less common, sexually transmitted diseases.

†Salvarsan and other heavy metals employed in the standard treatment of syphilis prior to the use of penicillin in the 1940s were highly toxic and might have done more harm than good from the point of view of individuals treated with them. (Cf. Louis Lasagna, The VD Epidemic, pp. 60-61, 65-66.

problem more serious, quantitatively and as a matter of concern to the state. The program then established remained substantially unchanged until World War II. Local authorities were required to set up free treatment centers; physicians were provided with free diagnostic facilities and free arsenical drugs for treating their private patients; maternity and child welfare clinics, and midwives, became involved in the detection and prevention of venereal disease. These measures were carried out under earlier public health legislation, but, with the aim of protecting the public, a new law, the Venereal Diseases Act of 1917, prohibited unqualified treatment or private advertising of remedies. From the distribution of the drugs provided free for treatment of syphilis, it appeared that the great majority of known syphilis cases received treatment through the local authority centers.(1) The program was about 75 percent financed by the central government, and administered from its beginning through World War II by Colonel L.W. Harrison. The thrust of the British approach was to make treatment as freely and readily available as possible. It eschewed anything that might discourage the patient from seeking and continuing treatment, including cost, compulsion, reporting, and case finding.(2)

World War I also saw a burst of activity in the United States. Clinics opened with Red Cross funds and later with federal support, provided under the Chamberlain-Kahn Act of 1918. The United States Interdepartmental Social Hygiene Board was another product of that legislation, as was the Division of Venereal Diseases in the U.S. Public Health Service. The Draft Act of 1917 and many state laws during and after the war provided for the repression of prostitution and the closing down of "red light" districts. In 1912 the Army had established a control program involving compulsory prophylaxis, physical inspections, punishment, and early treatment. In the war General Pershing insisted on the enforcement of these measures, and on keeping American soldiers out of French brothels. State laws, based on a model developed by the Public Health Service, required physicians to report cases to the local public health officer, and to report again if the patient deserted treatment. These state laws also provided for modified isolation, or compulsory segregation if necessary, of infectious cases, and for clinics for the indigent or medically indigent, as well as for free laboratory work and drugs.(3)

While the wartime program continued in Britain with little change for 20 years, there was a falling off of governmental interest in the interwar period in the United States, where federal funds were cut drastically in 1920 and eliminated altogether in 1926. Incidence and prevalence of venereal diseases, especially gonorrhea, cannot be determined with any confidence, because of problems of diagnosis, lack of reporting, and so on, but it seemed that in Britain syphilis was on the decline and gonorrhea was fairly constant.(4) In the United States, emphasis on reporting was at least in part responsible for a rising rate of reported cases, especially of syphilis.(5) (The increase was blamed on inadequate control measures and the reemergence of red light districts.) In Britain, prostitution, which was not illegal, seemed to to be on the decline.(6)

The experience of World War I, and the rise in known cases as mobilization advanced, provided another strong impetus to the expansion of British and American state intervention to control venereal disease, before and during World War II. New laws and regulations were enacted, treatment facilities and preventive measures were greatly expanded, case finding and education developed, and government-sponsored research produced important advances in treatment and prevention.

In the United States, the revival of interest in venereal disease control began several years before World War II. Thomas Parran, the Surgeon General of the Public Health Service from 1936, had studied venereal disease control in Europe. He admired the free and universal treatment facilities in Britain and the consideration with which patients were treated, but regretted the lack of reporting, case finding, and compulsory treatment, all of which were employed in the Scandinavian countries. His article, "Why Don't We Stamp out Syphilis?" appeared in Reader's Digest, with a circulation of 2 million in 1936.(7) The following year he published a very influential book, Shadow on the Land: Syphilis. He called a conference on venereal disease control in Washington at the end of 1936, and stimulated a strong revival of active control programs in the States, fueled in part by federal funds for public health under the Social Security Act. Congress provided specific funding for state control programs in 1938, through the National Venereal Disease Control Act (LaFollette-Bulwinkle).

War's approach sustained the control movement, gave it urgency and a wide base of support. Harry S. Mustard, Director of Columbia's School of Public Health, reflected in 1945:

> Like the enthusiasm of 1918, the present wave of interest arose to some extent out of war psychology or preparation for war, when it is easier to obtain an appropriation of a million dollars than it is ordinarily to get one of a thousand. Encouraging, however, is the fact that whereas previous interest in venereal diseases was limited to a relatively small group of experts, the present interest has a much broader base and rather remarkable public support.(8)

Parran followed up Shadow on the Land with another popular book, Plain Words about Venereal Disease, co-authored by Assistant Surgeon General R.A. Vonderlehr. The book is dedicated to General John J. Pershing and gives central place to syphilis and gonorrhea as the "prime wasters of manpower" and hence "saboteurs" of the national defense.(9)

In many respects, then, syphilis and gonorrhea represented problems similar for the state to those associated with tuberculosis. Both became more serious in wartime and elicited a similar state response in the two countries. There are important differences, however, which are essential to an understanding of the different patterns of control developed in Britain and the United States.

Many diseases, including tuberculosis, and perhaps all illness, have some stigma attached to them, but the case of venereal disease was unique, because of its close connection with sexual behavior. Venereal disease was seen not simply as a medical or public health matter, but as a moral question. It was a symptom of, a punishment for, a warning against, sexual immorality. Control of syphilis and gonorrhea was an aspect of the social control of sexuality. Ideology, therefore, played a crucial role in shaping efforts at controlling these diseases, even where manpower and military-economic efficiency needs dictated that the efforts be made. Important differences between the two countries in the degree and nature of state intervention in this area require explanation at the ideological level.

An even greater threat to military efficiency than tuberculosis, venereal disease is unique in that infection of a soldier is almost always caused by contact with a civilian.(10) (The obvious exception, homosexual contact between soldiers, was little discussed.) It is also true, of course, that armies often spread venereal disease among the civilian populations of countries they occupy, through rape and the destruction of means of livelihood other than prostitution, which was the experience of Vietnam, for instance. But that was not the situation in Britain or the United States, and was not in any case the perspective in which venereal disease appeared as a problem for the state. Soldiers also spread venereal disease among those with whom they had unforced, noncommercial sex, including casual acquaintances and spouses. But the state's concern was with the soldiers' efficiency, not with the health of the women they infected, except insofar as they then became a source of further infection of the military.

Sex, and with it venereal disease, presented a peculiar aspect of the relationship between the state's military apparatus and the civilian population. Military efficiency seemed to require efforts to limit or regulate sexual contact with civilians. Civilian-military relations, then, take on a greater and quite different significance for venereal disease control than is the case with tuberculosis.

THE MORAL QUESTION: MAKING FORNICATION SAFE

The "Conspiracy of Silence"

At the time of the International Conferences for the Prophylaxis of Syphilis and Venereal Diseases, held in Brussels in 1899 and 1902, venereal disease was a taboo subject in both Britain and America. It was not discussed in polite society, was not mentioned in speeches, in the press, or in the schools. There was general ignorance about symptoms and prevention, and no effective treatment. Although it reached epidemic proportions,* physicians did not treat it epidemiologically: they did not, that is, try to trace contacts, isolate the infectious, or recommend prophylaxis, and there was no immunization.(11)

The taboo on public discussion was strong in both countries, and constituted a major obstacle to control of these diseases. The reformers, those physicians, clergymen, social workers and others who wished to extend the public health movement to this area, faced what they called a "conspiracy of silence."(12) As syphilis and gonorrhea ravaged the armies of World War I, and arsenical compounds seemed to offer effective treatment of syphilis, the taboo weakened. Silence and ignorance persisted, however: in the mid thirties, syphilis was still seldom discussed in the press and never mentioned on the radio. That there was no lack of interest in the subject is suggested by the strong demand for the issue of Reader's Digest containing Parran's 1936 article, a demand that permanently established the mass circulation of the magazine in England. In the United States, it prompted the press to abandon its traditional silence.(13)

Behind the taboo was a more general reticence, rooted in religious and moral attitudes, about sex as a matter for public discussion. Chastity provided adequate protection against these diseases, so that falling victim to them was a result of, and a punishment for, sin. Its prevalence among the poor and the foreign-born was further evidence of their moral as well as social inferiority. Only as a rare scandal did these diseases afflict members of respectable society, according to this view.(14)

These attitudes persisted unevenly in the late thirties, and have not disappeared in the early 1980s. Parran's lead was not followed with uniform enthusiasm, even among physicians and public health officers. Massachusetts public health leaders, Nels A. Nelson and Gladys L. Crain, noted in 1938:

> Among the rank and file of health officers, however, there has been a considerable feeling of resentment that the

---

*Parran and Vonderlehr estimated in 1941, "whether labeled or not, it is probable that every family in America has suffered some loss from syphilis or gonorrhea, either directly or indirectly, either in this generation or the last" (Plain Words, p. 16). They may well have exaggerated, but their statement is suggestive of a level of concern, if not quite panic, felt and communicated by the American advocates of strong state action.

control of any diseases as "indecent" as these should be considered a public health problem. Not all physicians cheerfully accept the suggestion that the treatment of the infected, without prejudice, is a proper function of the medical profession. Innumerable hospitals deny admission to those unfortunates who are known to have gonorrhea or syphilis. It has annoyed many health officers to have to provide treatment at public expense for those "prostitutes" or otherwise "sexually promiscuous" persons whose infections "label them for what they are." The aid of the police is still too readily sought when a person stops treatment prematurely or when there is a problem in epidemiology to be solved, thus fostering the idea that to be infected is to be guilty of a crime.(15)

"Enlightened" reformers shared, to a greater or lesser extent, the underlying assumptions of those they criticized. They pointed out, for example, that a large proportion of infections, especially of wives and children, were "innocent," implying that those acquired in the course of illicit sex were guilty.(16)

Prophylaxis

The question of prophylaxis was an especially difficult one for the reformers. Rubber sheaths were issued as prophylactics to troops in World War I, but many clergy and others, who were sympathetic to the venereal disease control movement, objected to this approach. Some opposed mechanical prophylaxis because it was a form of birth control. But chemical prophylaxis, the application of some compound of silver, mercury, and other substances after exposure to infection, was also controversial. In Britain the movement split over this question; a new organization formed, the Society for the Prevention of Venereal Disease, which advocated prophylactic methods not accepted by the older National Council for Combating Venereal Diseases (later the British Social Hygiene Council).(17)

The threat of venereal disease was, or seemed, a powerful deterrent to sexual license. To provide people with the means to indulge in sexual promiscuity without fear of infection tended to encourage immorality. It was the "guilty," after all, who would, premeditating their sin, take advantage of such measures. The mainstream of the British movement, fearful of estranging the sympathies of its moralist and religious wing, made a curious distinction in the interwar years between "prophylaxis" (i.e., prevention), which they did not countenance, and "early preventive treatment" (i.e., prophylaxis), which they advocated. That is, they disapproved of prophylactic kits, which would enable people to disinfect themselves after exposure to infection. On the other hand, they urged that "those who have succumbed to temptation should at once repair to . . . a clinic and receive early preventive treatment, i.e., be disinfected."(18) The distinction between disinfecting oneself and going to a clinic to be disinfected, between "prophylaxis" and "early preventive treatment," rested on the amount of premeditation that was thought to be involved. "A reversal of this policy," argued Sir Malcolm Morris in 1919, "by affronting the moral feeling of the country and antagonizing the Churches, would, in my opinion, be disastrous."(19)

Such thinking persisted in World War II. It was not the basis of government policy in either country, and especially not in the armed forces. But it was a source of outside pressure and criticism, to which the military had to respond. At a conference convened by the Central Council for Health Education, the Ministry-of-Health-sponsored body that took over responsibility for venereal disease propaganda work in World War II, the Archbishop of Canterbury, Dr. Temple, objected to the preventive, public health thrust of government policy in these terms, as The Times reported:

> In the Army instruction was given in the use of prophylactics. The implication was that the authorities expected a considerable number to practice fornication.
>
> The root trouble was the treatment of what was primarily a moral problem as if it were primarily a medical problem. The fundamental objection to Regulation 33B (a wartime control measure discussed below) was the same − its very existence tended to create the suggestion that infectious contacts were being dealt with and the concern of the Government was to make fornication medically safe. What was primarily a moral problem with a medical aspect was being treated as if it were primarily a medical problem with a moral aspect.(20)

Leading American clergy raised similar objections to official policy, especially that prevailing in the armed forces. Like the Archbishop of Canterbury, they emphasized the need to instruct soldiers in the duty and necessity of chastity. That was the proper, as well as the most effective, prophylaxis.(21)

Social Hygiene vs. Public Health

Venereal disease control was always the main focus of the social hygiene movement, but its supporters saw such control as an aspect of the regulation of sexual behavior in general. Like unmarried motherhood, prostitution, sexual promiscuity, perversion, and sex crimes, syphilis and gonorrhea were "symptoms" of poor social hygiene, or poor "sexual adjustment." Social hygienists sought to improve sexual behavior through preventing and repressing prostitution, rehabilitating prostitutes and other sexually "delinquent" females, through the provision of wholesome recreation, and through changing social conditions that fostered sex delinquency. Prominent among the latter were saloons, gambling, and the sale of alcohol.

This emphasis on disease control through the social control of sexual behavior was much more pronounced in the United States than in Britain or other European countries. Indeed, social hygienists led and shaped the American anti-venereal-disease movement, in part because of the reluctance of public health officers to take responsibility for this area of disease control. Thomas Parran played a major role in bringing about a change of approach in the 1930s, a shift toward a public health definition of the problem as one of communicable disease control. He argued that about three-quarters of venereal disease was not transmitted by prostitutes, and that where a decline in incidence had taken place, as in Sweden, Britain, Massachusetts, or Wisconsin, it had nothing to do with higher morals or improved sexual behavior. An efficient public health disease control program, not moral instruction or exhortation, reduced syphilis and gonorrhea.(22)

Parran did not argue for eliminating moral improvement as an approach to disease control, but he relegated it to a relatively minor role. He saw venereal disease in precisely the terms to which Archbishop Temple objected, as "primarily a medical problem with a moral aspect." Nels Nelson led a move, successful in several state public health departments, to substitute "genitoinfectious" for the judgmental term "venereal." He thought that Parran's approach had succeeded in lifting the lid of censorship in the United States because it talked about disease control rather than sex behavior, and so was less offensive to American prudery.(23) But he also warned against wholesale rejection of social hygiene. Though much broader in objective and scope than the control of two prevalent communicable diseases, social hygiene might be necessary to sustain any improvement. Morality was an aspect of preventive medicine. Public health measures had led to improvements in the control of tuberculosis, for which there was no effective immunization or treatment, but could not have been successful without concurrent improvements in standards of living, nutrition, housing, and so forth. In the same ways gains in the control of genitoinfectious diseases could be maintained "only if there is some concurrent improvement in the sexual habits of our people."(24)

Thus Nelson (and co-author Crain) sought to bring about a rapprochement between the social hygienist and the health worker. "The one finds in the prevalence of gonorrhea and syphilis an excellent argument for better sexual behavior. The other may discover that better social hygiene will be the 'preventive medicine' through which gonorrhea and syphilis will be <u>kept</u> under control some time in the future."(25)

Nelson's argument, like Parran's work, reflects the powerful pressure exerted by the social hygienists and the need to placate them. It also reveals, unintentionally, the deep ambivalence in the attitude of the moral crusaders to disease control. For, if the prevalence of venereal disease is an "excellent argument for better sexual behavior," to reduce it without the need for moral improvement (e.g., by prophylaxis, or the development of a vaccine) is to weaken the case for sexual morality. Social hygiene and disease control, morality and health, were in principle separable, and some public health workers argued for the elimination of moral concerns. For the present, however, they shared common ground. Both seemed to point in the direction of repressing prostitution.

THE CRUSADE AGAINST PROSTITUTION

Britain

A continuing argument had gone on through the nineteenth and twentieth centuries, in Europe and America, about whether it was better to license and regulate prostitution, or to repress it. Britain did neither. Contagious Diseases Acts of 1864, 1866, and 1869 had subjected women near military and naval bases to medical examination if suspected of being infectious, and to hospitalization if found to be so. These laws were bitterly opposed, as unconstitutional and discriminatory against women, as amounting to state regulation, and hence recognition, of prostitution.(26) Parliament repealed the acts in 1886, and thereafter passed no laws that could be construed as regulating prostitution. Free clinics for the treatment of venereal disease, established during and after World War I, were available to prostitutes and anyone else, but there was no compulsion. The public health policy, from World War I on, was to make treatment as easily available as possible. Any form of compulsion was considered undesirable, as tending to discourage people from disclosing their infection and seeking treatment. Clinics encouraged patients to notify their contacts and advise them to seek examination and treatment, but there was no system of reporting or case finding. Prostitution itself was not an offense, but soliciting was punishable under vagrancy laws, while living on the immoral earnings of another and keeping a brothel were illegal.(27)

World War II produced an increase in state activity to control venereal disease, but not an effort to repress prostitution. The number of free treatment centers was greatly expanded, and the Ministry of Health launched an unprecedented health education program, using a radio broadcast, nearly 4,000 large advertisements in the press, two films, a national conference, photographic exhibitions, and some 160,000 posters. It was "the most intensive effort in the field of health education yet undertaken in this country."(28) One result was an increase in numbers seeking examination and treatment at clinics, and a rise in the proportion of those found to be free from infection. Another was the breaking down of the taboo on the subject, a process furthered by debates in both Houses of Parliament and an extensive correspondence in The Times.

Partly as a result of American pressure, the British government did take a temporary, wartime step in the direction of case finding and compulsory treatment, with the promulgation of Defence Regulation 33B. This measure resulted from a need to bring "under treatment a number of girls and women who were responsible for much inefficiency through venereal infection of service men."(29) It provided that any person reported by venereal disease practitioners as being suspected of having infected two or more of their patients might be compelled to undergo examination and treatment as necessary until free from infection. The regulation, and American example, stimulated contact tracing. Many local authorities used social workers to find and persuade people (the overwhelming majority were female) reported under the Regulation. These workers also persuaded voluntary patients to get their contacts to come for examination, followed up patients who discontinued treatment prematurely, and expended "much effort on removal of social difficulties which are often responsible for premature discontinuance of attendance."(30) Two official committees, one of them including American and Canadian military representatives, examined the question of widening the scope of compulsion to a general system of notification and compulsory treatment. Both decided against it.

These measures, though they resulted in 82 prosecutions, did not amount to a crackdown on prostitution. In general, prostitution appeared a relatively minor source of infection, compared with noncommercial sexual activity, and there was no widespread move to make it illegal or increase police harrassment, at least until after the war. Dr. Edith Summerskill argued in Parliament that 33B was inadequate and discriminatory, a position that had some support in Britain, but much more in the United States.(31)

The United States

The contrast with the American approach to prostitution and venereal disease could not be more striking. Although Parran estimated that only a quarter of the incidence of syphilis and gonorrhea resulted from prostitution, he gave strong emphasis to its repression in Shadow on the Land. In Plain Words, published four years later (in 1941), he and Vonderlehr argue still more forcefully for attacking prostitution. The earlier book's defensiveness, a response to criticism that he gave too little weight to repressing prostitution, is replaced by an aggressive advocacy of stronger action. In stressing this aspect of venereal disease control, Parran appealed to a crusading spirit of moral reform, which was less interested in controlling disease than in attacking vice.

Moral reformers seldom felt it necessary to argue for the connection between repressing prostitution and controlling venereal disease. It was widely assumed that most infections were caused by prostitutes. The Army's Surgeon General, in supporting legislation to prohibit prostitution near military bases, claimed that three quarters of all venereal infections in the Army could be traced to prostitutes.(32) Surveys conducted by the American Social Hygiene Association (ASHA) itself during the war tended, with localized exceptions, to suggest that soldiers acquired the large majority of their infections from "pick-ups" and girl friends. A bill introduced in the New York State legislature, making it an offense for an infected person to have sexual intercourse with a serviceman or -woman, included the comment that "investigation has shown that four times as many soldiers are infected from contact with willing girls in their teens as from prostitutes."(33) This did not deter social hygienists from thundering against those who favored regulating rather than repressing prostitution (a view that was privately held more than it was publicly advocated at this time). They argued that regulation did not work as a public health measure, but assumed that another approach to prostitution, their own, was the key to controlling venereal disease.*

War gave a fresh impetus to the flagging antiprostitution forces. In the 1920s and 1930s, ASHA's research on prostitution conditions in the United States had revealed "in many places throughout the country a backward trend not only in conditions, but in public thought and action concerning them."(34) Red light districts had returned, and politicians showed little interest in providing funds or active support for repression. In some cases they were influenced by the "racketeers" who organized the prostitution. War gave renewed force and urgency to the reformers' arguments, the drift and tone of which are illustrated in the following paragraph by Jean B. Pinney, of ASHA, addressed to a receptive audience, the readers of Social Service Review.

---

*Subsequent research indicated that the individual's risk of infection from intercourse in a medically controlled brothel with ablution facilities was very small — .03 percent in one study (F. Ray Bettley, "The Medical Conduct of a Brothel"; see also the comments by Douglas J. Campbell, "Venereal Diseases in the Armed Forces Overseas" and T.E. Osmond, "Venereal Disease in Peace and War"). ASHA and U.S. Army propaganda, on the other hand, implied that infection was all but inevitable.

Social workers need no argument to convince them that the "racket" of commercialized prostitution is an ugly scar on the national countenance — a dragging ball-and-chain on human progress. This sordid business is seen to be an injustice, since it victimizes one group of human beings for the dollar-profit of others; a subversive element, since it traps and soils our youth and undercuts our family life; and a menace to the public health, since it is a chief means of spreading the dangerous infectious diseases of syphilis and gonorrhea. Because of this latter fact particularly, while prostitution in peacetime is like some treacherous underground stream slowly washing away the solid earth, in times of national crisis like the present, unless firmly curbed, it may become like a raging torrent, damaging the health and morale of our armed forces and of workers in industry to an extent affecting the war's outcome.(35)

Pinney calls her article "How Fares the Battle Against Prostitution?" and the war image recurs throughout. ("Crusade" would have been a more accurate, if less topical, metaphor, since the struggle was more protracted than a battle, and had religious overtones.) While the upper levels of the federal government took action along the lines advocated by ASHA, there was some resistance and foot dragging at the local level. Reformers usually blamed such reluctance to fight vice on the influence of organized crime. "(A)ll of us are realizing anew that we must fight side by side and shoulder to shoulder," said Pinney. "Especially while the battle is joined with the powerful and slippery prostitution racketeers."(36)

But many ordinary people were ambivalent about trying to eradicate prostitution. They held some informal version of the functionalist theory of prostitution expounded in sociological terms by Kingsley Davis and others.(37) That is, prostitution, far from undercutting family life as Pinney believed, actually functioned to preserve it by providing the "naturally promiscuous" male with an extramarital sexual outlet, or safety valve, which did not threaten to usurp the wife's role. Furthermore, prostitutes took the pressure off "respectable" young women, enabling them to keep their virtue while their future husbands satisfied their lust elsewhere. If soldiers were denied access to prostitutes, they would seduce, or even rape, the other young women of the town. "The young soldier on leave, with healthy instincts, is quite likely to seduce a 'good girl' if there is no 'bad girl' around or if one is too difficult to find."(38) A naval surgeon, Winfield Scott Pugh, expressed in 1941 a common argument for regulated brothels: "What substitute do we offer for prostitution? Like it or not, somebody's daughter."(39) The prostitute herself was not, in this sense, anybody's daughter; she was outside the sphere of respectable society, but necessary to its respectability. As

Greek democracy had rested upon slavery, so bourgeois respectability depended upon prostitution.

More feminist and less benign interpreters of these social arrangements noted that their functioning rested on a split between sensual (prostitute, mistress) and sentimental (wife, mother) in men's relations with women, on a double standard, which resulted in the brutal exploitation of some (lower class) women, the sexual deprivation of most, and the oppression of all. Wilhelm Reich, one of the most influential exponents of this view, argued that this split, "together with the linking of sensuality and monetary gain, results in a complete degradation and brutalization of love life, its most important repercussion being widespread venereal diseases, which, also unintentionally, become an essential part of the conservative sexual order." Venereal disease was, in his view, "the practical counterpoint of marital morality and the ideology of chastity."(40) A corollary of the popular-functionalist view of prostitution (as safeguard of female virtue) was, as Reich argued, that one way to reduce prostitution was to facilitate the entry of young women into sexual life.

Despite the lack of general enthusiasm for a crusade against prostitution, the reformers succeeded in persuading the federal government to pursue the repression of prostitution as a matter of national defense. In May 1940, an Eight-Point Agreement on venereal disease control emerged out of meetings between the War and Navy Departments, the Federal Security Agency (to which the Public Health Service reported), state health departments, and ASHA. The agreement between the governmental bodies, supported by ASHA, formed the basis of civil-military collaboration and included active support for the repression of prostitution.(42)

"It comes as a surprise to many otherwise well-informed persons," wrote Pinney, "to learn that nearly all states have laws of some type which can be used effectively to curb prostitution and that twenty-two states now have legislation which, if conscientiously enforced, could entirely deprive the prostitution racketeers of their profit and power."(43) These laws had fallen into disuse, but now the federal government joined the moral reformers in pushing for their enforcement. Following the Eight-Point Agreement, a Division of Social Protection was established in the Federal Security Agency. Its main task was to implement Point Six of the Agreement, which called for the repression of prostitution.

The Social Protection Division collected information about the extent of prostitution in local communities, and inquired about what control measures, from supervision of bars to rehabilitation of prostitutes, were being carried out. Police chiefs and sheriffs set up the National Advisory Policy Committee on Social Protection, and the American Bar Association established a National Committee on Courts and Wartime Social Protection, to advise and work with the division. Field representatives of the Social Protection Division tried to stimulate and coordinate local activities. They encouraged measures to supervise hotel and bar operations, to control pimping by taxicab drivers, and to rehabilitate and redirect prostitutes. In their zeal, they often antagonized other agencies involved in controlling prostitution and venereal disease, gave advice to local and state health authorities that was in conflict with Public Health Service recommendations, and were belligerent in their approach to the armed services.(44)

A year after the Eight-Point Agreement, in May 1941, federal pressure for repression of prostitution increased as a result of passage of the May Act. Under this law, prostitution within a reasonable distance of a military or naval establishment became a federal offense. The act stimulated local law enforcement efforts, with the threat that federal agencies such as the FBI would intervene if they failed to take adequate measures. It was invoked only twice, in Tennessee and in North Carolina, but it proved an effective lever with which federal agencies, in collaboration with ASHA and other voluntary organizations, could move reluctant local agencies into action.(45)

Another expression of the state's concern at the national level was the Interdepartmental Committee on Venereal Disease Control, which was established in December 1941, upon the impetus of Parran's and Vonderlehr's book, Plain Words About Venereal Disease. It brought together in a series of meetings leading representatives of the Army, Navy, Public Health Service, and Federal Security Agency, and also, in an advisory capacity, members of other governmental and voluntary agencies, such as the Justice Department and ASHA. It discussed problems of cooperation among different agencies at the local level, and the desirable extent of federal intervention. At its third meeting there was a split over how the May Act should be used. Parran of the Public Health Service and William F. Snow of ASHA supported invoking the act in several test cases, as a way of impressing the "underworld." The military services and the Federal Security Agency, concerned about conflicting jurisdictions and relationships with state and local agencies, thought the act should be invoked only if local forces proved clearly unable to deal with the situation.(46)

There is no doubt that the antiprostitution program produced results; the problem is in interpreting them. All over the country, in over 600 cities and towns, red light districts closed down between 1940 and 1943. In some areas closing of brothels was associated with a decrease in known venereal disease rates, in other areas there was no clear relationship.(47) In January 1945, Walter Clarke voiced ASHA's concern that red light districts would return, venereal disease would increase, and government funding would dry up, once the war was over.(48) By the early 1950s, writers in the Journal of Social Hygiene were noticing (in different articles) an upward trend in prostitution and a decline to their lowest points ever of the incidence of syphilis and gonorrhea.(49) Even during the war, as the brothels closed, the reformers' attention turned increasingly to the clandestine (unorganized) prostitutes, and to the far more numerous "victory girls" or "cuddle bunnies" – the young teenage girls who were seen as aggressively promiscuous and willing to sleep with any man in uniform.(50) It became increasingly difficult to ignore the very great extent to which sex took place outside marriage and prostitution.

Although repression of prostitution was a prominent part of American social hygiene activities, there were many other aspects of the venereal disease control program. The number of clinics rose from 1,222 in 1939 to 3,088 in 1941, and in 1942 the first rapid treatment centers opened, with funds provided under the Lanham Act legislation providing federal aid for areas affected by the war.(51) These centers, administered by the Public Health Service, were able, with new advances in treatment and the beginning use of penicillin, to reduce the time of treatment from months or years to 10 days for syphilis, and to a few hours for gonorrhea. The Public Health Service and ASHA both carried on very extensive educational efforts, using films, posters, literature, and meetings, Contact tracing improved, the Public Health Service (as well as the Army and other agencies) sponsored research into all aspects of venereal disease control, and many states introduced modified laws requiring blood tests for syphilis as a condition of receiving a marriage license and as a part of prenatal care.(52)

Britain and the United States

Many observers noted the difference in approach between Britain and the United States. The official American view, as expressed by Parran and the U. S. Army, was that the British traditionally considered sex as a private and personal matter, in which the state had no business. Their individualism was such that they would not countenance state compulsion in private sexual relations with a prostitute or anyone else (so long as they did not create a public nuisance), or in notification, case finding, or treatment. "As far as contacts are concerned, the patient is encouraged to bring his wife and children in for examination, or to tell his paramour that she is responsible for his infection. If he does not, that is his business, says Colonel Harrison – and no concern of the government!"(53)

This is unlikely to be a wholly adequate explanation, since, if anything, individualism and hostility to government were stronger and more tenacious in the United States. A more popular and less diplomatic view found expression in the columns of Newsweek and Time. Unlike the U. S. Army, they saw prostitution as more widespread in Britain than almost anywhere. Thus, Time told its readers,

In the practice of the world's oldest profession, the water fronts of Port Said or Shanghai have never hummed more briskly than do London's Piccadilly and gaudy, shoddy Soho. Day and night girls walk their dogs, soliciting. Police look the other way. . . .(54)

"VD in London, Battle of Piccadilly Circus Among the Army's Worst" was the title of one of Al Newman's reports for Newsweek.(55) Prostitution flourished, they argued, because British prudery inhibited public discussion and a serious confronting of the problem. This explanation is also doubtful. Prudery certainly characterized British attitudes to discussion of matters pertaining to sex, but probably not more so (or not much more so) than was the case in the United States. These journalists based their interpretation on highly selective data – Piccadilly Circus and Soho were not representative. In the U. S. Army view, according to its medical historians, prostitution, especially of an openly organized variety, was less of a problem in Britain than in the United States, and the higher incidence of venereal disease among GIs in Britain was almost entirely a result of easily available, noncommercial sexual relationships.(56)

An alternative approach would be to look at the peculiarities of American, rather than British, society. The American drive against prostitution had much of the character of a moral crusade, like the temperance movement. Prohibition and the repression of prostitution may both be seen as products of a greater American willingness to enforce morals through legislation and policing, and a greater optimism about the possibilities of moral reform as an aim of social policy. This may in turn reflect a higher degree of social heterogeneity, with weaker informal controls. Repressing prostitution had been one way in which progressive reformers of the business and professional classes hoped to elevate and improve the lives of the urban immigrants. The United States, furthermore, had strong puritan religious and theocratic traditions on the one hand, and lacked the lingering British aristocratic tradition, an ideology contemptuous of bourgeois moralism and zeal, on the other. Certainly, the continuing difference in approach to heroin and other drug addiction – repression in the United States, free supply combined with treatment under the National Health Service in Britain – suggests that the contrast in approach to official social control of deviant behavior, or moral improvement through state coercion, persists, is far-reaching, and extends beyond the sphere of sexual relations.

Sexual repression was, in Freud's view, the necessary basis of civilization; for Reich it was essential to the reproduction of capitalist social relations. Whatever the general truth of these ideas, the notion that controlling sexuality is especially crucial to holding society together is deeply and widely believed, especially by those who fear that it is in danger of flying apart. (The Moral Majority is only the most recent organized expression of the belief that sexual license threatens the social fabric.) In the United States, the ethnic, cultural, religious, political, social, and regional hetero-geneity that accompanied mass immigration and the rapid growth of industries and cities made that fear especially strong, above all among those native middle-class strata whose social position was most threatened by the transformation.(57) The need to hold society together in the face of disintegrative forces seemed greater in the United States than in Britain, and "social hygiene," including the repression of prostitution, seemed vital to the task.

Reichian hopes and moralist fears about the political conse-quences of the sexual revolution may have been exaggerated or misplaced, as recent changes in sexual mores suggest.(58) But the conviction on which they were based, that sexual repression was necessary to the maintenance of the social order, was widely held. The historical context of that belief in the United States favored organized social intervention and legal coercion, as opposed to reliance on informal mechanisms of social control. War posed a less objectively compelling threat to the American social order than the British, and health and manpower needs were not as pressing. But in the case of venereal disease control, unlike nutrition or tuberculosis control, the war tapped a reservoir of crusading moral interven-tionism in the United States. Despite the obstacles it put in the path of prophylaxis, that tradition was useful to those, above all in the Army, who had an interest in controlling venereal disease. It enabled them to obtain higher priority for their activities within the U. S. Army than their British counterparts could achieve, and it supported the repression of prostitution, which they thought necessary on public health grounds.

NOTES

(1)   PEP (Political and Economic Planning), Report on the British Health Services, pp. 289-92.

(2)   Thomas Parran, Shadow on the Land, pp. 111-21.

(3)   Nels A. Nelson and Gladys L. Crain, Syphilis, Gonorrhea and the Public Health, pp. 210-17. See also Harry S. Mustard, Government in Public Health, pp. 160-62; Parran, Shadow, pp. 69-88; Parran and R. A. Vonderlehr, Plain Words About Venereal Disease, pp. 67-77.

(4)   PEP, British Health Services, pp. 290-92; Sydney M. Laird, Venereal Disease in Britain, pp. 32, 71.

(5)   Monroe Lerner and Odin W. Anderson, Health Progress in the United States, pp. 179-81.

(6)   Mrs. C. Neville Rolfe, "Sex-Delinquency, " New Survey, pp. 296-300.

(7) Reader's Digest 29 (July 1936), pp. 65-73

(8) Mustard, Government in Public Health, p. 161.

(9) Parran and Vonderlehr, Plain Words, pp. 1, 48.

(10) Ibid., p. 81; Vonderlehr, "As the United States Public Health Service Sees It," Journal of Social Hygiene 26 (1940), p. 415.

(11) Parran, Shadow, pp. 25-26.

(12) Sir Malcolm Morris, Story of English Public Health, p. 135; Nelson and Crain, Syphilis, Gonorrhea, pp. 1-5; Vonderlehr and J. R. Heller Jr., The Control of Venereal Disease. On the persistence of the "conspiracy of silence" into the 1930s, see Parran, Shadow, pp. 224-30. For a review of the literature from the turn of the century to the late 1930s, see Harvey J. Locke, "Changing Attitudes Toward Venereal Diseases," American Sociological Review 4 (1939): 836-42. See also Lasagna, VD Epidemic, pp. 118-41.

(13) Parran, Shadow, p. 120; Nelson and Crain, Syphilis, Gonorrhea, p. 1.

(14) Parran, Shadow, pp. 73-74.

(15) Nelson and Crain, Syphilis, Gonorrhea, p. 2.

(16) Ibid., p. 2; Parran and Vonderlehr, Plain Words, p. 9.

(17) W. M. Frazer, History of English Public Health, p. 345.

(18) Morris, Story of English Public Health, pp. 139-40.

(19) Ibid. Sir Malcolm Morris was a member of the Royal Commission on Venereal Diseases, and of the Executive Committee of the National Council for Combating Venereal Diseases.

(20) The Times (February 27, 1943), p. 2.

(21) U. S. Army, Preventive Medicine, vol. 5, p. 196. Cf. Gene Tunney, "Bright Shield of Continence," pp. 43-46. For the contrary view, against continence, for a strictly medical approach, including all other methods of prophylaxis, and for the toleration and control of prostitution, see Harry Benjamin, "Morals Versus Morale."

(22) Parran, Shadow, pp. 119, 207, passim; Parran and Vonderlehr, Plain Words, pp. 38-41.

(23) Nelson and Crain, Syphilis, Gonorrhea, p. 6.

(24) Ibid., p. 7.

(25) Ibid., p. 8.

(26) Judith R. Walkowitz, Prostitution and Victorian Society.

(27) C. H. Rolph, Women of the Streets, pp. 15-44, 61-75, 112-116.

(28) U. K. Ministry of Health, On the State of the Public Health During Six Years of War, p. 250.

(29) Ibid., p. 70.

(30) Ibid., p. 71.

(31) "Great Britain: 33B and a Prayer," Time 40 (December 28, 1942): 23-24. Cf. on the weaknesses of 33B: U. S. Army, Preventive Medicine, p. 237.

(32) U. S. Army, Preventive Medicine, p. 142.

(33) Quoted by Benjamin, "Morals Versus Morale," p. 186. For opinions of the proportion of venereal disease transmitted by

prostitutes, see Eleanor Lake, "Trouble on the Street Corner: Brass Buttons and Junior Misses — A Headache for All Society," Common Sense 12 (May 1943): 147-49; Bascom Johnson, "When Brothels Close, VD Rates Go Down," Journal of Social Hygiene 28 (1942): 525-35; Richard A. Koch, "Promiscuity as a Factor in the Spread of Venereal Disease," ibid. 30 (1944): 517-29; Walter Clarke "Teamwork in Venereal Disease Prevention," ibid. 30 (1944): 107-27 (esp. p. 117); Benjamin, "Morals Versus Morale," pp. 185-87 and the sources cited there. Extreme variations in estimates probably reflect, as Benjamin suggests (p. 186), both vagueness in the definition of "prostitute" and emotional predispositions of the investigators. The more scientific studies indicated that prostitution was a relatively minor factor in the transmission of venereal disease in Britain and the United States, but was much more significant in some other countries, such as Japan. See R. R. Willcox, "Prostitution and Venereal Disease: Social Considerations of Prostitution"; idem, "Prostitution and Venereal Disease: Proportion of Venereal Disease Acquired."

(34) "Milestones in the March Against Commercialized Prostitution," Journal of Social Hygiene 27 (1941): 430.

(35) Jean B. Pinney, "How Fares the Battle Against Prostitution?" p. 224.

(36) Ibid., p. 225.

(37) Kingsley Davis, "Prostitution," in Robert Merton and Robert Nisbet, ed., Contemporary Social Problems, New York: Harcourt, Brace & World, 1961, pp. 262-88. Cf. Ned Polsky, Hustlers, Beats, and Others, Chicago: Aldine Publishing Co., 1967, pp. 186-202.

(38) Benjamin, "Morals Versus Morale," p. 195.

(39) Quoted in ibid., p. 195.

(40) Wilhelm Reich, The Sexual Revolution, pp. 35-36, 45. For useful recent discussion of Reich, see Paul Robinson, The Freudian Left; Juliet Mitchell, Psychoanalysis and Feminism; Bertell Ollman, Social and Sexual Revolution.

(41) See Reich's comments on Judge Ben Lindsey in Sexual Revolution, pp. 98-99.

(42) U. S. Army, Preventive Medicine, pp. 140-41; Pinney, "How Fares?" pp. 238-39.

(43) Pinney, "How Fares?" p. 239.

(44) Ibid., pp. 232-35; U. S. Army, Preventive Medicine, pp. 162-66. See also the statement of Eliot Ness, Director of the Division of Social Protection: "Division of Social Protection Announces Program," Journal of Social Hygiene 27 (1941): 433-35. On the role of the police, see Charles S. Rhyne, "The War Program and Prostitution," American City 57 (1942): 109-11.

(45) U. S. Army, Preventive Medicine, pp. 174-79; Eliot Ness, "Prostitution, Social Protection and the Police: The New Offensive

Along the Police Front," Journal of Social Hygiene 28 (1942): 365-71.

(46) U. S. Army, Preventive Medicine, pp. 167-68; "Relationships in Venereal Disease Control of the Army and Navy, the U. S. Public Health Service, the Office of Defense Health and Welfare Services, and the American Social Hygiene Association," Journal of Social Hygiene 29 (1942): 100-5.

(47) Johnson, "When Brothels Close," Journal of Social Hygiene 28 (1942): 525-35; "A 'Second Front' Against Prostitution," Report of Special Committee on Enforcement of the National Advisory Police Committee, Journal of Social Hygiene 29 (1943): 43-50; Harry P. Cain, "Blitzing the Brothels" ibid., 29 (1943): 594; Agnes E. Meyer, Journey Through Chaos, pp. 111-19; U. S. Army, Preventive Medicine p. 173.

(48) Walter Clarke, "Postwar Social Hygiene Problems and Strategy," Journal of Social Hygiene 31 (1945): 4-15.

(49) E.g., Norman R. Ingraham, Jr., "National and International Problems in the Control of Venereal Disease," Journal of Social Hygiene 37 (1951): 123-29; Paul M. Kinsie, "Prostitution — Then and Now," Journal of Social Hygiene 39 (1953): 241-48.

(50) Meyer, Journey Through Chaos, pp. 114, 109-10; U. S. Senate, Wartime Health and Education, pp. 6-7, 84-100, 263; Richard Lingeman, Don't You Know There's a War On? pp. 101-5; Lake, "Trouble on the Street Corner," Common Sense 12 (May 1943): 147-49; Koch, "Promiscuity," ibid. 30 (1944): 517-29 (see note 33 above).

(51) Parran and Vonderlehr, Plain Words, p. 32; Lucia Murchison, "Rehabilitation in Action," Journal of Social Hygiene 30 (1944): 298-301.

(52) George Gould, "Does Your State Need New Social Hygiene Laws?" Journal of Social Hygiene 28 (1942): 536-47; idem, "Twenty Years' Progress in Social Hygiene Legislation," ibid. 30 (1944): 456-69 (the entire November, 1944 issue, vol. 30, no. 8, including Gould's article, is devoted to "A Review of Principles and Progress in Social Hygiene Legislation"); Eleanor Shenehon, "News from the States and Communities," ibid., 31 (1945): 460-63.

(53) Parran, Shadow, p. 116.

(54) Time 40 (December 28, 1942), p. 23.

(55) Newsweek 21 (June 14, 1943), p. 60.

(56) U. S. Army, Preventive Medicine, p. 242.

(57) Richard Hofstadter, The Age of Reform; Joseph R. Gusfield, Symbolic Crusade.

(58) Michel Foucault, The History of Sexuality, vol. I, p. 131.

8

VENEREAL DISEASE CONTROL: THE ARMY AND SOCIETY

The contradictions of a social formation, it has been said, take on an intense and concentrated form in its army.(1) The variety of conflicting and ambivalent attitudes we have examined in the society as a whole existed within both British and American armies, as well as imposing contradictory pressures on them from without. The army's primary policy objective was to maintain military efficiency by reducing to a minimum the incidence of venereal disease in the armed forces. But how was it to be achieved, and how were the demands of morality and morale (the latter certainly vital for fighting ability) to be satisfied at the same time?(2)

Some favored moral exhortation to chastity, with punishment for those who rendered themselves unfit for service as a result of their fornication. They believed that purity was the only perfect prophylaxis, and also favored it on principle, while disapproving other forms of prophylaxis as inducements to immorality. Others, with or without deference to the moralists, favored a more strictly medical approach, emphasizing screening, easy and early treatment without punishment or moralizing, and all kinds of prophylaxis. Some wanted to repress prostitution primarily on moral grounds, others mainly as a public health measure. Some wanted to close the brothels and encourage chastity in the interests of discipline and morale, as well as for health and moral reasons; others supported prostitution or other sexual outlets as important for morale.

Civilian attitudes to the army were also contradictory and ambivalent. The soldiers were "our boys," fighting our fight and serving the nation in its time of need. For some women and teenage girls, that consideration enhanced the attractiveness of servicemen, making sex almost a patriotic duty.(3) For many of an older generation, it brought home the obligation to protect the servicemen from exploitation, and, in the words of Woodrow Wilson's World War I pledge on behalf of the federal government, to ensure that "the men committed to its charge will be returned to the homes and communities that so generously gave them with no scars except those won in honorable conflict."(4) At the same time soldiers appeared not only as our sons in uniform, but also as sexual marauders who threatened our daughters' virtue and safety. As one GI put it in a letter to a former professor:

> I never realized it would make so much difference when I was in uniform. You would think I had leprosy. In spite of a lot of patriotic platitudes – it's all different. You have your choice between a low level of sensual woman who is always about where men in uniform are and who isn't exactly a prostitute but isn't much better, and the very professional welfare-conscious attache of the USO. There isn't anything else. My buddy and I got a big laugh out of a newspaper comment that people near army camps were opening their homes to soldiers on Sundays. The truth is that most of them live in mortal fear that one of their "innocent" daughters might be contaminated by a date with one of the boys in uniform.(5)

The notion of prostitution as functional for respectable society appeared in concentrated form in the sphere of civilian-military relations. Prostitutes and other "bad girls" on the one hand, and the USO on the other, formed a shield to protect the "nice girls" by deflecting the soldiers' libido into either vice or wholesome recreation.

These attitudes and conflicts characterized both societies and both armies, but are most interestingly explored in terms of the U.S. Army's relations with civilian branches of the American state and the voluntary social hygiene movement on the one hand, and with the British state and society on the other. Some 1.5 million GIs were stationed in Britain in the latter part of the war, and about another half million were there for short periods while in transit.(6) The U.S. Army attempted to carry out a consistent policy of venereal disease control at home and in Britain, and faced a different combination of forces in each case. In examining the attempt we can bring out both the similarities and differences of the two countries' social policies in this area, as well as their interaction.

THE U.S. ARMY: POLICY AND PRACTICE

Repression of organized prostitution was central to the War Department's policy for the control of venereal disease. General Pershing had strongly insisted on this policy in the Great War, even making fitness for command conditional upon conscientious efforts to carry it out. His General Order 77 not only carried that warning to commanders, but also put brothels out of bounds to the American Expeditionary Force (AEF), surrounded them by military police, stopped the sale of hard liquor, and required vigorous measures for the prophylaxis and treatment of venereal disease.(7)

The order resulted from a report to Pershing by Dr. Hugh M. Young, chief of the venereal disease department for the AEF, about conditions at St. Nazaire, France. Troops passing through that small port had an exceptionally high rate of infection. Young recalled:

> The city was inadequately policed by the M.P., crowded with grog shops, and maintained six houses of commercial prostitution. I found many drunken soldiers on the streets and queues several blocks long leading to the houses of prostitution, where the inmates entertained from 50 to 65 men each in the afternoon and evening.(8)

This image, of men rendering themselves unfit for service by the thousand, deeply influenced military police with regard to venereal disease control. In World War II, as we have seen, the army collaborated with other governmental and voluntary agencies to prevent such a situation. It was party to the Eight Point Agreement of 1940, and cooperated with the Public Health Services, ASHA, and later the Social Protection Division of the FSA. The army was represented on the Interdepartmental Committee on Venereal Disease Control and National Advisory Venereal Disease Committee. It argued for and supported the May Act at home and tried to prevent contact with prostitution abroad (by persuading civil authorities to close down brothels or by using military police to keep soldiers out). It cooperated with the Public Health Service in its contact tracing and separation programs.

Despite its official position, the army was constantly under pressure from outside critics, and had some difficulty persuading civilian agencies involved in the antiprostitution campaign that it took the problem seriously. Even after several years of top-level collaboration, which increased as mobilization developed, the two top administrators of the Public Health Service, Parran and Vonderlehr, launched a strong attack on the army in their Plain Words About Venereal Disease. Not only was policy carried out very unevenly at lower levels of command, they said, but there was also lacking the firm, forceful leadership from top military commanders and from the secretaries of the War and the Navy that had been present in the first World War. Their most critical chapter had the pointed heading, "Wanted — Another Pershing, Another Baker" (Newton D. Baker had been Secretary of War during World War I). The book caused a temporary rift in the generally cordial relations between the army and the Public Health Service, but its wider effect was to stimulate a more coordinated and active response, by military and civilian agencies, to prostitution and venereal disease.(9)

In practice, the War Department always had difficulty in getting its policy carried out by commanders in the field. Many of them tolerated or supported prostitution. They favored regulated red light districts, with medical inspections, rather than repression, as a venereal disease control measure. In 1940, word reached the War Department and the Army's Surgeon General that army medical officers were in some areas of the United States examining prostitutes as a protective measure to safeguard soldiers from venereal disease. In 1941, a series of letters and directives was fired off, from the Adjutant General and the Chief of Staff to all commanders, and from the Surgeon General to surgeons of major headquarters. Their message was that the army's position was in danger of being misunderstood, with the result that it would, and already had, come in for severe criticism. Commanding officers were directed to encourage local officials to enforce laws repressing prostitution and not to permit in any circumstances personnel under their control to "make inspections of any character of houses of prostitution."(10)

As the army moved into other theaters of operation, the unevenness with which official policy was implemented became more pronounced. Further directives issued from the headquarters of the European theater (ETOUSA). They included a letter, issued at the end of 1943, from the commanding officer to each unit commander: based on Pershing's General Order 77, it linked fitness for command to the percentage of physically fit soldiers.(11) In May 1944, a month before D Day, ETOUSA headquarters issued the following directive:

> The practice of prostitution is contrary to the best principles of public health and harmful to the health, morale, and efficiency of troops. No member of this command will, directly or indirectly, condone prostitution, aid in or condone the establishment or maintenance of brothels, bordellos, or similar establishments, or in any way supervise prostitutes in the practice of their profession or examine them for the purposes of licensing or certification. Every member of this command will use all available measures to repress prostitution in areas in which troops of the command are quartered or through which they may pass.(12)

Two months later, when the Chief of the Preventive Medicine Division visited Cherbourg on July 6, 1944, exactly a month after D Day, he found conditions strongly reminiscent of those described by Dr. Young at St. Nazaire a quarter of a century before:

> There he found, in Cherbourg, houses of prostitution being run for, and indirectly by, U.S. troops, with the familiar

pattern of the designation of one brothel for Negro troops and the others for white, with military police stationed at the doors to keep order in the queues which formed.(13)

The Cherbourg brothels were placed off limits almost immediately after this situation was reported, but similar problems arose as American troops swelled the population of Paris. There the provost marshal for the area, apparently on orders from the commanding general, "made a tour of Paris brothels . . . for the express purpose of selecting certain houses of prostitution to be set aside for officers, others for white enlisted men, and still others for Negro enlisted men."(14)

PROPHYLAXIS IN THE ARMY

Unlike civilian agencies, the army placed very great emphasis on prophylaxis. It made condoms available at post exchanges and later distributed them free through medical supply channels. Soldiers were instructed and encouraged in their use. Chemical prophylaxis was widely available throughout the army, either at prophylactic stations or in the form of individual kits. It had drawbacks – the procedure was complicated and prolonged, required the use of more than one ointment, and often involved irritation and pain – but the army tried to overcome these by extensive chemical research. It produced a new single-ointment prophylactic which did not irritate, burn, or stain, called PRO-KIT. (It substituted sulfathiazole-calomel for Protargol-calomel.) However, the war was over before these improvements were widely available, either in individual kit form or at prophylactic stations. The army also experimented with oral administration of sulfathiazole for gonorrhea prophylaxis and used it widely in the last two years of the war.(15)

In this area of venereal disease control, there was no foot-dragging in the army. Indeed, in many cases, commanding officers resorted to compulsory methods of distributing prophylactic materials. The army's Surgeon General opposed this practice, which was severely criticized by civilians, including clergy and politicians. But he vigorously defended the official policy of making prophylaxis widely available and encouraging its use.(16)

Religious and other civilian leaders criticized this policy as encouraging promiscuity and as in conflict with the educational program, which stressed continence and the dangers of venereal disease. The Surgeon General replied that moral aspects of venereal disease were important, but the interests of military efficiency required that it be treated as any other disease. Since a certain, unknown, proportion of men were going to expose themselves to infection no matter what advice they received, it was important to make prophylaxis readily available for all. The War Department assured its critics that it recognized that continence was "the only perfect method of preventing venereal diseases" and that "for moral and physical reasons it is in favor of chastity among troops."(17) But it would not rely solely, or very heavily, on what Gene Tunney in Reader's Digest called the "bright shield of continence" to protect its military manpower.(18)

The official policy on chastity was probably taken even less seriously at lower levels of command than that on prostitution. One sergeant stationed in Britain allegedly advised his men one morning at reveille, "I'm told that we've got thirty thousand rubbers in the supply room. I want you people to do something about this."(19)

THE U.S. ARMY IN BRITAIN

American soldiers in Britain were symbols of money, sex and power. As such they attracted in concentrated form the admiration and bitterness, gratitude and resentment that the British reserved for their wealthier, more potent cousins. Commonalities of culture and language made "fraternization" much easier than in many other countries; but sharp, historical differences of attitude and policy made control of the venereal disease that resulted an exceptionally difficult and delicate undertaking.(20) The guest relationship of the foreign army to its allied host both facilitated friendly contacts between soldiers and civilians, and at the same time prevented the imposition of a single, coherent approach (the foreign army's) to venereal disease control. This proved not only one of the most difficult and complex public health problems of the war for the U.S. Army, but also a serious irritant in Anglo-American relations.

In addition to any intrinsic attraction men in uniform, engaged in a popularly supported war, may have had for young women, GIs in Britain had a special appeal. If they were sought after by American teenage "Victory girls," they seemed even more desirable to young English teenagers. As a British Home Office survey put it:

> To girls brought up on the cinema, who copied the dress, hair styles and manners of Hollywood stars, the sudden influx of Americans, speaking like the films, who actually lived in the magic country, and who had plenty of money, at once went to the girls' heads. The American attitude to women, their proneness to spoil a girl, to build up, exaggerate, talk big, and to act with generosity and flamboyance, helped to make them the most attractive boy friends. In addition, they 'picked up' easily, and even a comparatively plain and unattractive girl stood a chance.(21)

These perceived characteristics did not, of course, endear the GIs to other sections of the British public, among whom they were, according to Mass Observation, among the least popular foreign troops in Britain. They were, in the phrase of the time, "over-paid, over-sexed, and over here."(22)

GIs thus found it easy to have sexual relationships or encounters of a relatively noncommercial kind (their access to PX supplies, including nylons, certainly enhanced their appeal, however). Brothels such as those found in American red light districts or in France were almost unknown, and commercialized prostitution of any kind was not very common outside London and a few major cities. In these circumstances, infection of American soldiers in Britain with venereal disease arose very largely from friendly, nonprofessional sexual encounters.(23)

Time and Newsweek blamed the higher rate of infection among GIs in Britain than in the United States on rampant prostitution, but the British blamed high venereal disease rates among civilians on the presence of foreign troops, as well as on other social conditions favoring promiscuity. "Apart from the fact that country areas have been invaded by huge numbers of war workers and evacuees," observed the Ministry of Health, "families have been disrupted to a much greater degree than previously, and owing to the fact that the country has been a training ground and a base for the forces of other nations, besides our own, sexual promiscuity must have been prac-tised on a scale never previously attained in this country."(24) Concern over American soldiers with known venereal disease who were being sent to Britain developed in early 1944 to the point of becoming a diplomatic issue.(25) The increase in prostitution in wartime London was seen as a response to the effective demand of large numbers of well-paid American troops.(26)

In order to further official understanding of Anglo-American problems in this area, Dr. Joseph Earle Moore, chairman of the Subcommittee on Venereal Diseases, National Research Council, toured Britain in July 1943, consulting with military and civilian public health officials. His report noted American complaints of British failure to take or support serious control measures, including informational publicity and the repression of prostitution. He found that the English, on the other hand, objected not only to infected GIs being sent to Britain, but also to the "looseness" of American troops toward English women (a response to their provocativeness, according to his American informants).(27) Their high rate of pay, compared with that of British soldiers, led to increased sexual contacts — the bitterness of that complaint and its frequency reflected a popular resentment that went beyond concerns about health.

Black troops had a much higher incidence of venereal diseases than whites, and they were a special focus of British complaints.(28) Here too, professional and popular concern was not limited to health. It was also an expression of deep-seated British racism. As Moore reports it, the objection was that "Negro troops, because of their excessive sexual urge and the unfamiliarity of a certain small group of women with their social status, are a particularly potent source not only of venereal disease but of illegitimate pregnancies."(29) His recommendation in this regard was that "Negro troops in the ETO should be transferred to other theaters of operation, or alternately, their number held at its present level."(30)

In the special circumstances of wartime Britain, American medical officers found that much of their established approach to venereal disease control was not directly applicable. They could not attempt to further the repression of prostitution, as they did at home, by working with local law enforcement authorities. Such an approach would, they thought, have been seen by the British as meddling and ran counter to British law and policy, which tolerated prostitution "so long as the woman ostensibly was acting as a free agent, and so long as a procurer or facilitator was not readily apparent."(31) In any case, it was clear to the army if not to the journalists, that prostitution was a very small part of the problem.

The noncommercial character of most sexual encounters also affected the prophylaxis program. Soldiers were "much less impressed with the desirability or necessity of prophylaxis after exposure" when sex had been on a friendly rather than a commercial basis. The severe housing shortage also made it difficult to provide many ad hoc, off base prophylactic stations, while "British sensibilities forbade the display of prominent signs" to advertise the presence of those that were established, and the blackout prevented display of the usual green light at night. The prophylactic stations operated within the military installations, as part of every medical department, were, as always, much less popular. In the latter part of the war, the American Red Cross relieved the situation by providing space for prophylactic stations at its clubs. It was not until the end of 1942 that American-made condoms were available for GIs in Britain. The British supplies, though of good quality latex, were considered "totally unsatisfactory." "In the first place, they were too small, and, secondly, they were made with a deep constriction about 3 centimeters back from the closed end — the effect being to give them a freely hanging tip to which our soldiers objected strenuously."(32)

Though the U.S. Army did not attempt to establish a working relationship with the police, it did work on cordial terms with the Ministry of Health and with local medical officers of health. It also participated on the Joint Committee on Venereal Diseases with representatives of the British forces, the Ministry of Health, Home Office, and other government departments. At first the only control measure among the civilian population was the provision of free and easily available treatment, discreetly advertised in public lavatories. Public education, discussion, and publicity followed later, as well as a step toward compulsion in the form of Regulation 33B, which went into effect in November 1942. The Americans considered 33B inadequate, since it depended upon a complex procedure and required the complete name and address of the person identified. In the case of casual encounters between sexually highly active partners, that information was often not available.(33)

If the U.S. Army could not rely on standard American practices of reporting and contact tracing, they were nevertheless able to move some distance, and to push the British, in that direction. U.S. Army nurses, with the approval of the Ministry of Health and of the relevant local medical officers of health, engaged in contact investigations among the British civilian population in East Anglia. They approached nearly 500 women (well over half the total of twice-reported contacts for the whole country),(34) and told them that they might be in need of medical examination. The program was so successful that it influenced many British health officials to try similar schemes.(35) In general, though, the British procedure was, and remains, one of persuading patients to inform their contacts of possible infection and to encourage them to seek medical examination, rather than one of direct official approach to contacts.

CONCLUSION

Britain faced even more serious manpower problems than the United States, but in relation to venereal disease control the British state was far less interventionist. Often following the American lead, and responding to American example or pressure, it was less thoroughgoing and used less compulsion. The British army, like the American, abolished financial penalties ("hospital stoppages") for infection in order to encourage disclosure, placed brothels in foreign countries out of bounds to soldiers, provided prophylactic facilities, and issued condoms to its troops while in service abroad. The prophylactic stations, called early treatment ("E.T.") centers for reasons of moral tact, were on the military bases or camps, lacked privacy and, usually, warm water, and were little patronized. The higher levels of the British command tended to see venereal disease control strictly as a medical problem, to be left to medical officers. No General Pershing was either on hand or wanted, except by army medical personnel, who regretted the lack of support and leadership. It was characteristic that Regulation 33B was discontinued in Britain at the end of war, while the May Act became a permanent law in the United States.(36)

The exigencies of war pushed both states into stronger measures to control venereal disease than had prevailed in the 1930s, but they did not dictate the differences of extent and character of state action. Those differences reflected the distinct ideological structures, rooted in specific social histories, of the two nations.

As penicillin began to be used, and its application refined, in the treatment of syphilis and gonorrhea, those diseases rapidly lost their potency as threats to a nation's military and industrial strength. At the end of the war, high rates of infection were more than countered by ease and rapidity of treatment, so that noneffectiveness, or man days lost, due to venereal disease sank to record low levels even as incidence shot up.(37) After the postwar demobilization, incidence also declined and continued to do so until the late 1950s.(38) There was great hope that venereal disease would soon be conquered.

Such optimism was to prove misplaced. Government funding for venereal disease control was reduced in the 1950s as incidence declined. "As a disease control program approaches the end-point of eradication," an American public health official observed, "it is the program rather than the disease which is more likely to be eradicated."(39) As manpower ceased to be so urgently in demand, and ease of treatment and declining incidence rendered venereal disease a less serious threat to military or industrial efficiency, the programatic and research emphasis on prevention, pioneered, in spite of moral opposition, by the U.S. Army, lost ground. It was not until the 1970s, when venereal disease, and especially gonorrhea, reached epidemic proportions (more than double the highest levels of the 1940s), that public health officials again gave serious attention to prophylaxis. The women's health movement publicized what was known but little discussed, the preventive measures women could take in addition to insisting on use of a condom, from the army's technique of "short-arm" physical inspection of the male to vaginal prophylactics, such as Progonasyl and certain contraceptive creams, foams, and jellies.(40)

It also drew sharp attention to the discriminatory character of venereal disease control. From the Contagious Diseases Acts of nineteenth-century Britain through the control measures of World War II in both countries, women were treated as "hosts," sources of infection to be controlled. Most female sufferers were in fact wives who had been infected by their husbands. They had most to lose from the present gonorrhea epidemic, since they usually had no symptoms and so depended on being told they had been exposed to infection – something that did not reliably happen. Diagnostic tests were uncertain. Once venereal disease no longer robbed the military of large numbers of "man hours," and once men could get effective and convenient treatment for their easily recognized symptoms, prophylactic research and education were largely dropped, with devastating consequences for women.(41)

Exploration of the reasons for the current epidemic – such as changes in sexual mores, declining use of prophylactic methods of birth control, (e.g., condoms and vaginal creams) in favor of those that facilitate infection (the pill, intrauterine devices), the difficulty of diagnosing gonorrhea in women (the large majority of whom are asymptomatic in the early stages), and the emergence of dozens of penicillin-resistant strains of gonorrhea – lies beyond my present

purpose. It is striking, however, that in contrasting current literature on venereal disease control with that of the 1940s, one finds
the almost complete disappearance of any discussion of repressing
prostitution.

If changing sexual mores have affected patterns of infection,
they have also influenced thinking about control. Moralism and a
belief in social control of sexual behaviour as a means of disease
control have not disappeared, of course, but carry relatively little
weight among those involved in combating syphilis and gonorrhea.
"Making fornication medically safe" has become, not a damaging
accusation, so much as, expressed differently, a deliberate policy
goal. At a 1972 international symposium sponsored by the American
Social Health Association, successor of the social hygiene movement, a leading public health professor could call for closer cooperation with those involved in family planning in these terms:

> We are dealing with a common pattern of human sexual
> behavior, the results of which should be mediated in such a
> way as not to impair the health of those engaging in sexual
> activity but rather, permit them to carry on an activity
> which is normal and physiological, in such a way that disease
> transmission may be avoided and pregnancy may be wanted,
> rather than unwanted.(42)

World War II gave a strong impetus to the social hygiene
movement and to those moralists who could preach purity as a
matter of national defense, but it was also decisive in making
venereal disease control a matter of public health and not a moral
crusade. In the United States, ASHA won the battle against prostitution (at least, insofar as it closed down the red light districts), but
lost the war against promiscuity. Advances in treatment, made
during the war, may themselves have contributed to this outcome,
insofar as syphilis and gonorrhea now appeared readily curable
without hospitalization, and so lost most of whatever deterrent
force they might have had.

NOTES

(1) Leon Trotsky, History of the Russian Revolution, vol. 1, p.
252.

(2) Cf. Harry Benjamin, "Morals Versus Morale."

(3) Agnes E. Meyer, Journey Through Chaos, p. 114; Richard
R. Lingeman, Don't You Know There's a War On? pp. 101-2.

(4) Thomas Parran and R.A. Vonderlehr, Plain Words About
Venereal Disease, p. 67.

(5) Quoted in Lingeman, Don't You Know? pp. 104-5.

(6) U.S. Army, Preventive Medicine, vol. 8, p. 363.

(7) Colonel Joseph F. Siler, "Prevention and Control of Venereal Diseases," pp. 130-34; Parran and Vonderlahr, Plain Words, pp. 71-72.

(8) Ibid., p. 71.

(9) Ibid., ch. 4; U.S. Army, Preventive Medicine, vol. 5, p. 158.

(10) U.S. Army, Preventive Medicine, vol. 5, p. 142.

(11) Ibid., pp. 238-39.

(12) Ibid., p. 241

(13) Ibid., p. 243.

(14) Ibid., p. 246.

(15) Ibid., p. 200.

(16) Ibid., p. 202

(17) Ibid., p. 197.

(18) Gene Tunney, "Bright Shield of Continence."

(19) David Lampe, "Over Paid, Over Sexed, Over Here," Sunday Times Magazine, December 1966. Quoted by Angus Calder, People's War, p. 357.

(20) U.S. Army, Preventive Medicine, vol. 8, pp. 396-97.

(21) Sheila Ferguson and Hilde Fitzgerald, Studies in the Social Services, pp. 97-98.

(22) Lampe, "Over Paid," in Calder, People's War; Norman Longmate, The GIs; Calder, People's War, pp. 357-58.

(23) U.S. Army, Preventive Medicine, vol. 5, pp. 228-29.

(24) U.K. Ministry of Health, On the State of Public Health, p. 66.

(25) U.S. Army, Preventive Medicine, vol. 5, p. 238; ibid., vol. 8, p. 399.

(26) M.A. Wailes, "Social Aspect of Venereal Diseases," pp. 15-17.

(27) Moore's report is excerpted in U.S. Army, Preventive Medicine, vol. 8, pp. 399-401.

(28) Siler, "The Prevention and Control of Venereal Diseases," p. 93.

(29) U.S. Army, Preventive Medicine, vol. 8, p. 399.

(30) Ibid., p. 400.

(31) Ibid., vol. 5, p. 229.

(32) Ibid., p. 227.

(33) Ibid., p. 237.

(34) U.K. Ministry of Health, On the State of Public Health, p. 70.

(35) U.S. Army, Preventive Medicine, vol. 5, p. 238.

(36) On the British Army's response to the problems of venereal disease control, see F.A.E. Crew, ed., Army Medical Services: Administration, vol. 2, pp. 231-41; Sir Arthur S. MacNalty and W.F. Mellor, ed., Medical Services in War, pp. 84, 256-59, 271. See also S.C. Rexford-Welch, Royal Air Force Medical Services, vol. 1, pp. 399-404; Robert Lees, "Venereal Diseases in the Armed Forces Overseas (1)"; Douglas J. Campbell, "Venereal Diseases in the

Armed Forces Overseas (2)"; T.E. Osmond, "Venereal Disease in Peace and War."

(37)   U.S. Army, Preventive Medicine, vol. 5, pp. 331, 469-71.

(38)   J.D. Millar, "National Venereal Disease Problem," in International Venereal Disease Symposium, Epidemic, pp. 10-13.

(39)   Quoted by Lasagna, VD Epidemic, p. 4.

(40)   Boston Women's Health Book Collective, Our Bodies, Our Selves, 2d ed., New York: Simon & Shuster, 1976, pp. 169-71.

(41)   Gena Corea, The Hidden Malpractice, ch. 6; Edward M. Brecher, "Women — Victims of the VD Rip-Off," Viva, Oct.-Nov. 1973.

(42)   John C. Cutler, "Role of Prophylaxis and Education in Venereal Disease Control," in International Venereal Disease Symposium, Epidemic, p. 158.

9

CONCLUSION AND POSTSCRIPT

With manpower at a premium in all combatant countries, World War II made health a problem for the state as it had not been in the Depression. In the three areas we examined, nutrition, tuberculosis control, and venereal disease control, World War II elicited new levels of state activity in both Britain and the United States. The war was a more severe crisis for Britain, and produced a higher level of state intervention, in the areas of nutrition and tuberculosis control, as in other areas of health policy. Venereal disease control did not fit the pattern: it was an area of increased state action in both countries, but more so in the United States, even though it suffered a less acute manpower shortage.

For both countries, World War II constituted a crisis in which state and capital were vulnerable to an external, military threat on one hand, and to internal pressures from below (due to a compelling need for working-class labor, loyalty, and sacrifice) on the other. In response to these threats, the state acted authoritatively and relatively autonomously vis-a-vis the capitalist class, intervening in and organizing broad areas of economic and social life. Despite their suspicion of and hostility toward the state, capitalists were forced by the exigencies of war to submit to these statist, collectivist developments.

Social policy, therefore, was shaped by the state's need not only to ensure the fitness of the military and industrial manpower, but also to maintain national solidarity. It cannot be understood simply as the state's efforts to meet the objective need for a fit working and fighting population. Nor, on the other hand, is it very useful to see the evolution of health policy solely as a capitalist response to working-class struggle, in the manner of Vincente Navarro's recent study of the British health care system.(1) Both elements, in their interaction, were necessary to the outcome.

148

In World War II the heightened responsiveness of the British and American states to pressures from below resulted from the great shortage of labor and the need to mobilize fully the available human resources (including women and minorities) for the war effort. It reflected the state's dependence upon the loyalty, support, and self-sacrifice — as well as the industrial and military "manpower" — of the working class and other subordinate strata. A successful policy, then, would both protect the fitness of the working population and be an expression of the unity of the nation, without having adverse economic consequences. It would serve both efficiency and legitimation functions.

Pressure from below did not, of course, generally take the form of working-class, feminist, or minority mobilization in support of specific health policy demands. Even in its nutrition policy, state managers did not so much respond to organized working-class demands for food as they anticipated the potential impact of an inadequate or maldistributed food supply on hunger, food bills, and consequent unrest. Concern about the politically destabilizing effects of food shortages and inflation was, nevertheless, a potent element in the shaping of food policy, especially in Britain. In the United States, where the food supply problem was, together with the military situation, less serious, several food-related strikes prodded the state into responding more actively to workers' nutritional needs.

The state's concern with nutrition, as distinct from food, both reflected the need to maintain and reproduce a healthy population, and grew, as it were, spontaneously out of its responsibility for managing the total food supply. The British government, in particular, took ever more comprehensive control over what food should be imported and produced, and to whom it should go. As prewar food sources dried up, state officials and consultants argued for seeking the best nutritional value at the least expense, pushing policy beyond a strictly quantitative concern with supplies and prices.

If war imposed on the state system certain functional requirements, it did not thereby guarantee the capacity to meet them. There were indeed many obstacles in the way of developing a rational policy that simultaneously satisfied the demands of legitimacy and efficiency. One problem was that those demands tended to pull in different directions. The tuberculosis allowances scheme in wartime Britain illustrates the problems of pursuing a policy designed to protect the quality of the work force at minimum cost without regard to considerations of equity and humanity. It aroused bitter criticism and hostility, although, in view of the relatively small numbers of people affected, not on a scale to undermine seriously the legitimacy of the state. Fiscal economy and manpower were certainly the primary concerns, but even in those terms, of strict economic efficiency, the scheme was less than rational. It reflected conflicts of perspective between government departments and also, paradoxically, the pressure for a long-term conprehensive and coherent income maintenance policy.

If considerations of efficiency and legitimacy sometimes pointed in different policy directions, they were nevertheless inseparable. Efficiency in managing the economy and prosecuting the war were essential to the legitimacy of the state, and vice versa, as the period after Dunkirk, with its important social policy developments in Britain, attested.

Central to the state's difficulty in formulating and implementing social policy that serves the long-run interests of the national capital is the nature of the state system itself. Far from being a monolithic entity, or a cohesive actor, it reflects the contradictory, conflict-ridden, and even antistatist character of the capitalist class, while condensing, in Poulantzas's expression, the balance of class forces in the society within itself.(2) Politicians, of course, may be less immediately concerned with the efficiency or legitimacy of the economy and state than with getting elected. Voters judge administrations mainly on their economic performance, but individual legislators, especially in the United States, often represent primarily local and sectional interests. Congressional resistance to the wartime agricultural, food, and nutrition policies of the Roosevelt administration, from regulation of meat prices to the school lunch program, demonstrated the power of the agricultural sector within the state system itself. Divisions within the executive branch on agricultural matters reinforced the point.

War exposed and exacerbated the ineptitude of the legislature as an organ through which the state could carry out its task of being the cohesive factor in the society, while meeting the economic and military needs of the national capitalist class as a whole. It is precisely because the legislature is less autonomous in relation to particular capitalist interests that it is less able to act in the long-term general capitalist interest. The more the U.S. Congress appears, in Veblen's expression, as the "Soviet of Business Men's Delegates,"(3) 1) the less legitimacy it has as the factor of cohesion in the relations between classes, i.e., as representative of the nation and not just capital; and 2) the more the veto powers of particular elements of the capitalist class are likely to thwart the development of far-reaching policies and interventions necessary to ensure, under pressure, the long-term, general economic and political interests of the national capital as a whole. In short, the more conditions require the autonomization of the state vis-á-vis the capitalist class, the more they require the autonomization, growth, and dominance of the national executive. World War II, a more severe crisis for Britain, pushed this process farther there, where it was already more developed, than in the United States.

The fragmentation of the American state system puts (by design) severe limits on the national executive's ability to act decisively and coherently. That incapacity was a frequent source of frustration to the British and Canadian members of the three-nation Combined Production and Resources Board, and also contributed to the weakness of the Office of Price Administration. It was apparent in the conflicts and complexities of interagency and inter-governmental relations when it came to enforcing the May Act, an issue that divided the Public Health Service from the military. In its venereal disease control efforts, the U.S. Army not only felt the pressure of religious and voluntary organizations, but also the public criticism of the PHS's top officials, Parran and Vonderlehr. In the Army itself, despite its high level of centralization and clear chain of command, there were considerable difficulties in implementing an official policy that many high-ranking officers, as well as other ranks, did not take seriously.

In all three areas under study, the state drew upon the support and expertise of leading professional, and volunteers as it became more actively involved. State "intervention" in nutrition, tuberculosis control, or venereal disease control was not, then, entirely a matter of the state, as an impermeable body, moving into new regions. Rather, there was, to greater or lesser extent, a penetration of the state itself. As Shryock puts it in writing of the National Tuberculosis Association, its leaders "in effect infiltrated strategic federal centers concerned with tuberculosis control," guiding federal policy from within.(4) A similar process occurred with nutritional experts, although food policy was subject to other powerful considerations and their relative influence was correspondingly weaker. The American Social Hygiene Association played an important role in shaping government venereal disease policy, although more from without than within. Still, ASHA was routinely consulted and its advisory role was formally recognized in interagency meetings such as those that produced the Eight-Point Agreement and considered implementation of the May Act.

Where important interests, as opposed to concerns, are at stake, such permeation of the state system may fundamentally undermine the state's capacity to meet its efficiency and legitimation goals. The ability of professions and industries to use state regulatory bodies to serve, rather than limit, their immediate interests is well known. Medical influence on the development and operation of the National Health Service in postwar Britain suggests that we should think not simply of the state's taking over the health care system from outside, but also of doctors, to some degree, taking over the state. In the case of ASHA, however, the penetration of the state represented not the assertion of narrow professional interests and perspectives, but rather a vehicle for the transmission of cultural forces rooted in the country's social history. These forces stimulated a stronger American interventionism, which included pioneering research and prevention programs in the U.S. Army, but also limited and restricted it. They could no more be ignored, however, than the British could end the nutritionally useless practice of importing tea.

Many difficulties, then, constrain the state in its development of a rational health policy that ensures an adequate work force and military at minimum cost, while contributing to national cohesion, unity, and solidarity. It is not even clear, always, what such a policy would be, even if it could succeed politically and be implemented effectively. Apart from the problems of analysis and prediction, there are real conflicts of interest within the capitalist class, and between the state and the international character of capital, so that it may be hard or impossible to discern a national capitalist interest. Furthermore, what is necessary as a state response to pressure from below may have deleterious consequences for the economy, while what appears economically desirable may be politically dangerous.

Policies and programs that are functional at one time, economically or politically, may prove highly problematic in a later period (the U.S. social security program being only the most dramatic example). By then, however, they may have developed constituencies and expectations which make retrenchment or rationalization difficult to achieve. A brief look, by way of postscript, at the long-term impact of the health policy shifts wrought by the exigencies of war will suggest how some of the solutions adopted then contained within themselves the germs of present problems for the state and capital.

World War II gave way, not to the depression which people of all political persuasions expected, but to a quarter century of unprecedented growth, stability, and prosperity in all the major capitalist economies. A political and economic pax americana established the conditions for a rapid expansion of world trade, mostly between the advanced countries. The maintenance of wartime levels of arms spending sustained demand and absorbed a large part of the world's investable surplus, thereby evening out the boom-slump cycle of investment. Through its political, military, and economic activity the state, especially the American state, provided the basis for a period of expansion unparalleled in the history of capitalism. The problems and contradictions of this development were to emerge clearly by the late 1960s, but for two decades it appeared to many writers that capitalism had solved its basic problems, and that the state was central to the solution.

The crisis of world war was over. To the surprise of the onlookers, the patient had recovered and was stronger than ever. Capital had been forced to submit to the state's direction during the war emergency, but now the time had come to dismiss the doctor (whether he took the form of "Dr. New Deal" or "Dr. Win-the-War," to use Roosevelt's expressions). Controls and regulations were dismantled, rapidly in the United States, slowly in Britain.

But there was to be no return to the prewar order. The war itself had changed the world, shrinking it and interlocking its parts. If the American state established the rules and kept order, other states reorganized their national economies for competitive expansion and in defense against the American giant. In Britain, as in France, Italy, Germany, and elsewhere, important industries were nationalized or reshaped. With the increased scale of investment came a need to plan ahead, to ensure and predict transportation, supplies of raw materials, and labor costs. Capital, more than ever, needed a stable, predictable environment. It seemed to need, therefore, a positive interventionist state. The extent to which a state nationalized or reorganized its basic industries had more to do with the competitive strength of its national economy than with the ideological complexion of its government.

War had not only posed problems for the state that demanded new policy responses: it also seemed to solve some problems, at least temporarily. Unemployment, agricultural surpluses, and other features of the depression ceased to be problematic, and income maintenance withdrew from the center of the social policy stage. Health, on the other hand, became a vital concern in light of the state's urgent need for fit soldiers and workers. Out of the war came new levels of state expenditure and control in the health field – a comprehensive, universal National Health Service in Britain, new programs of federal funding for hospital construction and medical research and education in the United States.

The state pulled back, after the war, but not to its earlier position. A ratchet effect was evident, a common pattern where crisis elicits a new level of state interventionism, which in turn creates further economic and political effects preventing a return to the precrisis situation.

There has been no steady expansion of the state's role in social welfare provision. After the peak of the 1940s in Britain, there was a long stagnation and decline in provision, though not in expenditures. Universalist principles were compromised, and means tests multiplied. By contrast, a "private welfare state," of private pensions and health care plans, grew rapidly alongside the public systems. The crisis of war now past, there was a strong push toward "reprivatization"(5) of social provision, led intellectually by the Institute of Economic Affairs. In the United States the situation has been more complex. World War II produced major increases in state provision for veterans, but did not extend these benefits to the population as a whole. On the other hand, government policy with regard to wage controls and collective bargaining in a wartime period of labor shortage encouraged the growth of voluntary, job-related health and pension plans. The 1960s saw a new expansion of the state's role and autonomy, in response to new problems and pressures, themselves arising in part from changes in the structure of the labor force and the economy wrought by World War II.

But in both countries, the state's level of involvement in the health care system remained at a permanently higher level after the war. There had been a change in social consciousness, a shift in expectations of the government with regard to health, as there had been with regard to the functioning of the economy and the prevention of mass unemployment. The basis was being laid for the legitimation problems identified a quarter of a century later by political scientists and commentators who bemoaned the "revolution of rising entitlements" and the ungovernability of Western democracies.(6)

In other ways too, the solutions and adjustments of the war and immediate postwar period sowed the seeds of further contradictions and problems that would become more clearly apparent in later years. Government involvement stimulated the shift to hospital-based medical care administered by specialists. Many of the problems that now beset the American health care system – soaring costs, overspecialization and overuse of hospitals and surgery, lack of preventive and primary care, duplication of high-technology, low-utilization treatment facilities, and so forth – have their roots in government policies of the 1940s. These policies provided the financial underpinning for the growth of the medical empires of the 1960s and 1970s, by funding hospital construction, "heroic" medical research, specialist education. Public health, preventive policies, general practice, and other forms of ambulatory, nonspecialist care were neglected. Voluntary health insurance, encouraged as a fringe benefit by wartime wage controls, as well as postwar tax policy, often covered hospital care, but not office or home visits. Its cost-plus reimbursements provided security for the hospitals' investment in expensive technology. Many of these tendencies, for example hospitalization, specialist care, and technological intervention for low-risk childbirth, were already present before the war, but greatly accelerated in the postwar period.(7)

Despite the fears of its opponents, the British National Health Service proved a remarkably effective vehicle for controlling health care costs, since it enabled the state to determine the overall health budget. On the other hand, it has suffered from underinvestment, with old buildings and equipment, low wages for health workers, high turnover, and much dissatisfaction within the service. At the same time, compromises made in 1946, and government policy since then, have encouraged some of the same tendencies (which are, however, much less marked) as characterize American health care. The most significant problem the National Health Service has generated for the state, however, is its contribution to the politicizing of the economy. An important part of the social wage, it has been the target of government attempts to switch resources from consumption to investment by cuts and increased selectivity in social provision. As such, it has been part of the larger process described by Arthur Marwick as the "incredible shrinking social revolution" and the "withering away of the welfare state."(8)

In the 1940s the state became more heavily involved in health care because health had become an urgent concern for it, and because capital could not solve the problem on its own, through the market. One long-term result, however, was to make health care a locus of political conflict, to extend workers' struggles over living standards beyond the employer to the state. Despite the fragmented, apolitical, rank and file character of class conflict in the 1950s and 1960s (a shift in the locus of reformism where local, shop-floor struggles, not national unions or politics, were the key to advancing living standards), the basis was laid for a new generalization and politicization of class struggle. Shop-floor militancy could not defend the National Health Service, or other elements of the social wage.

In the United States, the state has become highly and increasingly involved in health-care financing, especially since the mid-1960s. Health has become more than ever a controversial political issue, but state involvement has not led to control over the costs of the system, rather the reverse. It has pumped new dollars into it. At the same time, large employers still have to meet heavy labor costs in the form of voluntary health insurance premiums, while consumers face substantial out-of-pocket expenses for health care.

The state's involvement in nutrition and in the control of tuberculosis and venereal disease illustrates many of the features of the larger pattern. They were all areas of concern and government action before World War II. The war made them urgent problems for the state, and elicited new levels of response. Capitalist resistance to an expanded or more autonomous state role weakened in the face of the crisis.

But each of these areas has a unique character and history. They are parts of a larger pattern, not miniature reproductions of it. Increased state intervention in the area of nutrition rapidly comes up against important capitalist interests, as well as being most directly a response to working-class pressure. That area, therefore, more closely resembles the big picture of which it is an element, than do tuberculosis and venereal disease control.

American state involvement in organizing the feeding of its people, we saw, never went as far as the British. The threat was less compelling, and the resistance of specific interests more effective. Rationing and price control quickly disappeared, but the National School Lunch Act of 1946 expressed a continuing commitment to ensuring minimum levels of nutritional adequacy. In this respect, the Employment Act of the same year was even more significant, as a symbolic expression and recognition of the state's responsibility to manage the economy so as to avoid a return to the mass unemployment and hunger of the 1930s. It was a political acknowledgement of new public expectations of the state, which would increasingly make effective economic policy central to a government's legitimacy. Hunger and malnutrition continued, of course, especially among the poor and minorities, and became a political issue in the 1960s, a decade which saw a major development of state involvement in the area of food and nutrition, including an extension of the school meals program and a new and massive food stamps program. These programs expanded greatly between the late 1960s and the mid-1970s.

In Britain, food controls were also dismantled, but it was not until 1954 that rationing was completely phased out. School milk and school meals became universally available. Nutrition was one aspect of the state's expanded social welfare role, one that had shifted substantially in a universalist direction, from rescuing the destitute to safeguarding decent levels of health, education, and security for the whole population. As part of the postwar welfare state, however, the welfare food programs that developed or greatly expanded in World War II suffered the same fate in the 1960s and 1970s as the welfare state in general. They took their place, alongside many other universalist programs, beneath the budgetary axe of successive governments. World War II, in this sphere as in others, set the pattern for the next quarter century or more. Later developments would all be either a consolidation of, or, especially after the first few years, a retreat from the welfare state principles established then.

Tuberculosis and venereal disease control do not have the same representative quality. War not only made these diseases immediate and urgent problems for the state. It also stimulated their solution. The diseases themselves persisted, although in the first postwar decade there was much optimism about their eradication. But they lost much of their terror for individuals, as a result of the ease and efficacy of medical treatment, and, in the case of tuberculosis, because of its rarity among all but the poorest sections of the population. More significantly, they lost much of their importance for the state and the economy as major drains of manpower. At the end of the war, as we noted, the incidence of syphilis and gonorrhea was rising in the American army, even as man days lost to those diseases were falling sharply. Government responsibility for tuberculosis and venereal disease control continued in the postwar years, but the character of the problems to which the state had responded in the war had largely changed.

In recent years the social policy solutions of the 1930s and 1940s, state responses to the crises of depression and war, have increasingly been blamed for the economic, political, and social difficulties of the present. The state is now the problem, not the solution. Both countries have elected antistatist governments committed to the partial reversal of policies and processes set in motion by earlier crises. Reprivatization, increased selectivity, and cutbacks of social programs, including health, have characterized the postwar period, especially in Britain, and are accelerating in pace in both countries. The extent to which the ratchet can really be filed down, and the growth and autonomization of the state reversed, remain to be seen. The next major social crisis, perhaps itself an outcome of present policies, will be a test.

NOTES

(1)   Vicente Navarro, Class Struggle, the State, and Medicine.

(2)   Nicos Poulantzas, Classes in Contemporary Capitalism.

(3)   Thorstein Veblen, Absentee Ownership, p. 47.

(4)   Richard Shryock, National Tuberculosis Association, p. 260.

(5)   Richard M. Titmuss, Social Policy, pp. 38-43.

(6)   See, for example, Daniel Bell, "Public Household," pp. 39-40; Anthony King, "Overload: Problems of Governing in the 1970s," Political Studies 23 (1975), pp. 162-74; Samuel Brittan, "The Economic Contradictions of Democracy," British Journal of Political Science 5 (1975), pp. 125-59.

(7)   Richard W. Wertz and Dorothy C. Wertz, Lying-In: A History of Childbirth in America, New York: Free Press, 1977, pp. 164-67.

(8)   Arthur Marwick, Britain in Century of Total War, pp. 389, 430.

BIBLIOGRAPHY

A. PRIMARY SOURCES

Altmeyer, Arthur J. et al. War and Post-War Social Security: The Outlines of an Expanded Program. Washington, D.C.: American Council on Public Affairs, 1942.

American City.

Anderson, Elin L. "Organizing the Community for Health Protection in Wartime." Public Welfare 1 (1945): 262-67.

Baker, Gladys Lucille. The County Agent. Chicago: University of Chicago Press, 1939.

Benjamin, Harry. "Morals Versus Morale in Wartime: The Sex Problem in the Armed Forces." In Victor Robinson, M.D., ed, Morals in Wartime. New York: Publishers Foundation, 1943.

Bennett, Hugh H. Soil Conservation. New York and London: McGraw-Hill, 1939.

Beveridge, William H. British Food Control. London: H. Milford, Oxford, Oxford University Press, 1928.

_____. Pillars of Security. London: Allen & Unwin, 1943.

_____. Social Insurance and Allied Services. London: H. M. S. O., 1942.

Birdseye, Miriam. Extension Work in Foods and Nutrition, 1923. Washington, D.C.: Government Printing Office, 1925.

Black, J. A. and Gibbons, C.A. "The War and American Agriculture." Review of Economic Statistics 26 (1944): 3-55.

Boudreau, Frank G. "Food for a Vital America." Survey Graphic 31 (1942): 128-29; 156-57.

Branscombe, Martha. "Reports from the Food Stamp Front." Social Service Review 15 (1941): 341-43.

British Medical Association. Nutrition and the Public Health: Medicine, Agriculture, Industry, Education. Proceedings of a National Conference on the Wider Aspects of Nutrition, April 27, 28, 29, 1939. London: British Medical Association, 1939.

_____. Committee on Nutrition (1933). Report of the Committee on Nutrition. London: British Medical Association, 1933.

_____. Committee on Nutrition (1947-50). Report of the Committee on Nutrition. London: British Medical Association, 1950.

Britton, Virginia. "The Cost of Food and the Adequacy of Income." Journal of Home Economics 29 (1937): 294-96.

Brown, Josephine Chapin. Public Relief 1929-1939. New York: Henry Holt & Co., 1940.

Burnham, John. Total War: The Economic Theory of a War Economy. Boston: Meador, 1943.

Calder, Ritchie. Carry On, London. London: English Universities Press, 1941.

_____. The Lesson of London. London: Secker & Warburg, 1941.

"Cato" (Michael Foot, Peter Howard, and Frank Owen). Guilty Men. London: Gollancz, 1940.

Churchill, Winston S. War Speeches, vol. 1. Edited by Charles Eade. London: Cassell, 1951.

Clark, F. Le Gros and Titmuss, Richard M. Our Food Problem: A Study of National Security. Harmondsworth, England: Penguin, 1939.

Colcord, Joanna C. Cash Relief. New York: Russell Sage Foundation, 1936.

_____."Stamps to Move the Surplus." Survey Midmonthly 75 (1939): 305-07.

Cole, G. D. H. and Cole, M. I. The Condition of Britain. London: Gollancz, 1937.

Combined Production and Resources Board (United States, Great Britain, and Canada). Impact of the War on Civilian Consumption in the United Kingdom, the United States, and Canada. Report of a special combined committee set up by the Combined Production and Resources Board. Washington, D. C.: Government Printing Office, 1945.

Crawford, Sir William and Broadley, H. The People's Food. London and Toronto: W. Heinemann, 1938.

Davis, Maxine. "Hungry Children." Atlantic Monthly 159 (January 1937): 83.

De Kruif, Paul. Kaiser Wakes the Doctors. New York: Harcourt Brace, 1943.

_____, in collaboration with Rhea De Kruif. Why Keep Them Alive? New York: Harcourt, Brace & Co., 1936.

Dos Passos, John. State of the Nation. Boston: Houghton Mifflin Company, 1943, 1944.

Drolet, Godias J. "Epidemiology of Tuberculosis." In Benjamin Goldberg, ed., Clinical Tuberculosis, vol. 1 Philadelphia: F.A. Davis Co., 1944, ch. 1.

Earley, James S., Hall, L. Margaret, and Berger, Marjorie S. British Wartime Price Administration, 1939-1943. Emergency Management Office, Office of Price Administration. Washington, D.C.: Government Printing Office, 1944.

Farson, Negley. Bomber's Moon. New York: Harcourt, Brace & Co., 1941.

Fishbein, Morris. The National Nutrition. New York: Bobbs-Merrill Co., 1942.

Fortune. "Death on the Working Front." A Supplement to Fortune 26, no. 1 (July, 1942).

Gold, Leon, Hoffman, A.C., and Waugh, Frederick V. Economic Analysis of the Food Stamp Plan. United States Department of Agriculture. A Special Report by the Bureau of Agricultural Economics and the Surplus Marketing Administration. Washington, D.C.: Government Printing Office, 1940.

Gollancz, Victor, ed. The Betrayal of the Left. London: Gollancz, 1941.

Halsted, Sophia. "The Nutritionist in a City Public Health Program." American Journal of Public Health 23 (1938): 850-51.

Hambidge, Gove. "Nutrition as a National Problem." Journal of Home Economics 31 (1939): 361-64.

_____. Your Meals and Your Money. New York and London: Whittlesey House, McGraw-Hill, 1934.

Harding, T. Swain. "America's Food Problem." Nation 152 (1941): 209-10.

Hart, P. D'Arcy and Wright, G. Payling. Tuberculosis and Social Conditions in England with Special Reference to Young Adults: A Statistical Study. London: National Association for the Prevention of Tuberculosis, 1939.

Heaf, F.R.G. and McDougall, J.B. Rehabilitating the Tuberculous. London: Faber & Faber, 1945.

Heseltine, Marjorie. "Nutrition Services in Maternal and Child Health Programs under the Social Security Act." American Journal of Public Health 28 (1938): 814-16.

_____. "The Nutritionist's Place in the Maternal and Child Health Program." The Child 2 (1938): 167-69.

Hilleboe, Herman E. and Kiefer, Norvin C. "Rehabilitation and Aftercare in Tuberculosis." Public Health Reports 61 (1946): 285-94.

Hopkins, Harry L. Spending to Save: The Complete Story of Relief. New York: W.W. Norton, 1936.

International Labour Office. British Joint Production Machinery. Montreal: International Labour Office, 1944.

_____. Workers' Nutrition and Social Policy. Studies and Reports, Series B (Social and Economic Conditions), no. 23, London: P.S. King for the I.L.O. (League of Nations), 1936.

Journal of Social Hygiene.

Katin, Zelma, in collaboration with Louis Katin. "Clippie": The Autobiography of a War Time Conductress. London: John Gifford, 1944.

Laird, Sydney M. Venereal Disease in Britain. Harmondsworth, Middlesex, England: Penguin Books, 1943.

Long, Catherine T. "Survey of School Lunch Legislation." Practical Home Economics 22 (1944): 258.

Long, Esmond R. "Tuberculosis and the War." Transactions of the National Tuberculosis Association. New York: N.T.A., 1944.

M'Gonigle, G.C.M. and Kirby, J. Poverty and Public Health. London: Gollancz, 1937.

Mackintosh, J.M. The Nation's Health. London: Pilot Press, 1944.

McLester, James S. "Nutrition and the Future of Man." Vital Speeches of the Day 2 (1936): 582-83.

Mason, Mary A. "Food and Nutrition in the FERA." Journal of Home Economics 27 (1935): 223-24.

Mass Observation. People in Production. London: Murray, 1942.

_____. "Social Security and Parliament." Political Quarterly 14 (1943): 245-55.

Meyer, Agnes E. Journal Through Chaos. New York: Harcourt, Brace & Company, 1943, 1944.

Morris, Sir Malcolm. The Story of English Public Health. London, New York, Toronto & Melbourne: Cassell & Co., 1919.

Municipal Yearbook.

Murrow, Edward R. This is London. Edited with an introduction, commentary, and footnotes, by Elmer Davis. New York: Simon & Schuster, 1941.

Mustard, Harry S. Government in Public Health. New York: The Commonwealth Fund, 1945.

Myers, J. Arthur. Man's Greatest Victory Over Tuberculosis. Springfield, Ill. and Baltimore, Md.: Charles C. Thomas, 1940.

National Association of Manufacturers. Industrial Health Practices. New York: N.A.M., 1941.

National Tuberculosis Association. Transactions of annual meetings.

Nelson, Nels A. and Crain, Gladys L. Syphilis, Gonorrhea and the Public Health. New York: Macmillan, 1938.

New International.

New Republic.

Newsweek.

Nicolson, Harold. Diaries and Letters 1939-45. Edited by Nigel Nicolson London: Collins, 1967.

Nourse, Edwin G. "The Economic Problem of Nutrition." Journal of Home Economics 30 (1938): 541-44.

_____. Marketing Agreements Under the AAA. Institute of Economics of the Brookings Institution Pub. 63. Washington, D.C.: Brookings Institution, 1935.

Ogburn, William Fielding, ed. American Society in Wartime. Chicago: University of Chicago Press, 1943.

Orr, John Boyd. Food and the People. London: The Pilot Press, 1943.

_____. Food, Health, and Income: Report on a Survey of Adequacy of Diet in Relation to Income, 2nd ed. London: Macmillan & Co., 1937.

_____. Nutrition in War. Based on an address delivered to a Fabian Society conference on food policy, February 1940. London: Fabian Society, 1940.

Orr, John Boyd and Lubbock, D. Feeding the People in Wartime. London: Macmillan, 1940.

Orwell, George. The Collected Essays, Journalism and Letters of George Orwell. Edited by Ian Angus and Sonia Orwell. Vols. 1-3. Harmondsworth, England: Penguin Books, 1970.

_____. The Lion and the Unicorn: Socialism and the English Genius. London: Secker & Warburg, 1941.

Parran, Thomas. "Outlook for Tuberculosis Control in the Civilian Population." Transactions. New York: National Tuberculosis Association, 1944, p. 144.

_____. Shadow on the Land: Syphilis. New York: Reynal & Hitchcock, 1937.

Parran, Thomas and Vonderlehr, R.A. Plain Words About Venereal Disease. New York: Reynal & Hitchcock, 1941.

Paterson, Robert G. "The Evolution of Official Tuberculosis Control in the United States." Public Health Reports 62 (1947): 336-41.

PEP (Political and Economic Planning). Report on the British Health Services: A Survey of the Existing Health Services in Great Britain with Proposals for Future Development. London: PEP, 1937.

Pilgrim Trust, The. Men Without Work. Cambridge: Cambridge University Press, 1938.

Pinney, Jean B. "How Fares the Battle Against Prostitution?" Social Service Review 16 (1942): 224-46.

Production and Marketing Administration. Food Consumption Levels in the United States, Canada, and the United Kingdom. Third Report of a Special Joint Committee set up by the Combined Food Board. Washington, D.C.: Government Printing Office, 1946.

Reed, Ellery, F. The Need of Casework in a Public Relief Agency. Chicago: American Public Welfare Association, 1938.

Reich, Wilhelm. Sex-Pol: Essays, 1929-1934. Edited by Lee Baxandall. Introduction by Bertell Ollman. Translated by Anna Bostock, Tom DuBose, and Lee Baxandall. New York: Random House, 1972.

_____. The Sexual Revolution: Toward a Self-Regulating Character Structure (1945). Translated by Theresa Pol. New York: Simon and Schuster, 1974.

Reid, Margaret G. Consumers and the Market. New York: F.S. Crofts, 1938.

_____. Food for People. New York: Wiley; London: Chapman & Hall, 1943.

Robinson, Victor, M.D., ed. Morals in Wartime. New York: Publishers Foundation, 1943.

Rolfe, Mrs. C. Neville. "Sex-Delinquency." In The New Survey of London Life and Labour, vol. 9: Life and Leisure. London: P.S. King & Son, 1935, pp. 287-345.

Rowntree, B. Seebolm. Poverty and Progress. London: Longman, 1941.

Siler, Col. Joseph F. "The Prevention and Control of Venereal Diseases in the Army of the United States of America." Army Medical Bulletin 67 (May 1943): special issue.

Smith, Charles. Britain's Food Supplies in Peace and War. A survey prepared for the Fabian Society. London: Routledge, 1940.

Smith, Charles. Food in Wartime. London: Fabian Society, 1940.

Smith Henry. Retail Distribution. London: Oxford University Press, H. Milford, 1937.

Snow, William Freeman. Venereal Diseases: Their Medical, Nursing, and Community Aspects. National Health Series edited by the National Health Council. New York & London: Funk & Wagnalls Co., 1924, 1937.

Sorenson, Helen L. and Gilboy, Elizabeth W. "The Economiocs of Low Income Diets." Quarterly Journal of Economics 51 (1937): 663-80.

Southworth, Herman M. "The Economics of Public Measure to Subsidize Food Consumption." Journal of Farm Economics 27 (1945): 38-66.

Speier, Hans. "Class Structure and Total War." American Sociological Review 4 (1939): 372-80.

_____. "The Effect of War on the Social Order." Annals of the American Academy of Political and Social Science 218 (1941): 87-96.

Stevens, Emily White. "Is There Too Much Food?" New Republic 76 (1933): 297-99.

Stiebeling, Hazel K. Are We Well Fed? A Report on the Diets of Families in the United States. Washington, D.C.: Government Printing Office, 1941.

Stiebeling, Hazel K., and Coons, Callie Mae. "Present-Day Diets in the United States." In U.S. Department of Agriculture, Food and Life: Yearbook of Agriculture 1939. Washington, D.C.: Government Printing Office, 1939, pp. 296-320.

Stiebeling, Hazel K. and Phipard, Esther F. Diets of Families of Employed Wage Earners and Clerical Workers in Cities. Washington, D.C.: Government Printing Office, 1939.

Stiebeling, Hazel K., and Ward, Medora M. Diets at Four Levels of Nutritive Content and Cost. Washington, D.C.: Government Printing Office, 1933.

Stiebeling, Hazel K., Monroe, Day, Coons, Callie M., Phipard, Esther F., Clark, Faith. Family Food Consumption and Dietary Levels, 5 Regions. Farm Series. Miscellaneous Publication No. 405. U.S. Department of Agriculture. Family Economics Division. Bureau of Home Economics. Washington, D.C.: Government Printing Office, 1941.

Stocks, Percy. "Vital Statistics of the Second Year of the War." Lancet 242 (1942): 189.

Survey Graphic.

Survey Midmonthly.

Sweezy, Maxine. Medical Care for Everybody? Washington, D.C.: American Association of University Women, 1945.

Thomson, H. Hyslop. Tuberculosis and Public Health. London: Longmans, Green & Co., 1920.

Time.

The Times. London

Tobey, James A. The National Government and Public Health. Baltimore, Md.: Johns Hopkins Press, 1926.

Tunney, Gene. "Bright Shield of Continence: Can The Grim Shadow of Venereal Disease be Lifted from our Armed Forces?" Reader's Digest 41 (August 1942): 43-46.

United Kingdom. Medical Research Council. Report of the Committee on Tuberculosis in War-time. M.R.C. Special Report Series No. 246. London: H.M.S.O., 1942.

United Kingdom. Ministry of Health. Advisory Committee on Nutrition: First Report. London: H.M.S.O., 1937.

United Kingdom. Parliament. House of Commons. Parliamentary Papers 1943-44. Statement on a National Health Service. London: H.M.S.O., 1944.

United States. Bureau of Human Nutrition and Home Economics. Consumer Purchases Study. Urban and village series. Washington, D.C.: Government Printing Office, 1939-41.

United States. Department of Agriculture. Agricultural Statistics. Annual. Washington, D.C.: Government Printing Office.

_____. Family Food Consumption in the United States, Spring 1942. Miscellaneous Publication No. 550. Washington, D.C.: Government Printing Office, 1944.

_____. Industrial Feeding in Manufacturing Establishments, 1944. Washington, D.C: Government Printing Office, 1944.

_____. Reports of the Secretary of Agriculture, 1939-1945. Washington, D.C.: Government Printing Office, 1939-1945.

United States. Department of Agriculture. Production and Marketing Administration. Food Consumption Levels in the United States, Canada, and the United Kingdom. First (Second, Third) Report of a special joint committee set up by the Combined Food Board. Washington, D.C.: Government Printing Office, 1944 (1945, 1946).

United States. Department of Labor. Bureau of Labor Statistics. Family Expenditures in Selected Cities, 1935-36. Vol. 2: Food. Bulletin no. 648. Washington, D.C.: Government Printing Office, 1940.

_____. War and Post-war Wages, Prices and Hours, 1914-23 and 1939-44. Bulletin no. 852. Washington, D.C.: Government Printing Office, 1945.

United States. Federal Emergency Relief Administration. Monthly Report of the Federal Emergency Relief Administration. Washington, D.C.: Government Printing Office.

United States. Federal Security Agency. Office of the Director of Defense Health and Welfare Services. National Nutrition Conference for Defense. First, Washington D.C., 1941. Proceedings of the National Nutrition Conference for Defense, May 26, 27, and 28, 1941. Called by President Franklin D. Roosevelt. Federal Security Agency. Office of the Director of Defense Health and Welfare Services. Washington, D.C.: Government Printing Office, 1942.

_____. Public Health Service. Annual Reports.

United States. National Research Council. The Food and Nutrition of Industrial Workers in Wartime. First Report. Reprint and Circular Series No. 110. Washington, D.C.: Government Printing Office, 1945.

_____. The Nutrition of Industrial Workers. Second Report of the Committee on the Nutrition of the Industrial Workers. Reprint and Circular Series No. 123. Washington, D.C.: Government Printing Office, 1945.

United States. National Resources Planning Board. Security, Work, and Relief Policies. Report of the Committee on Long-Range Work and Relief Policies to the National Resources Planning Board. Washington, D.C.: Government Printing Office, 1942.

United States. Public Health Service. Public Health Reports.

United States Senate. Wartime Health and Education. Hearings Before a Subcommittee of the Committee on Education and Labor, U.S. Senate, 78th Congress, 1st Session. Washington, D.C.: Government Printing Office, 1944.

Wailes, M.A. "Social Aspect of Venereal Diseases, Contact Tracing and Prostitute." British Journal of Venereal Diseases 21 (1945): 15-17.

Waller, Willard, ed. War in the Twentieth Century. New York: Dryden Press, 1940.

Wollman, Leo. Ebb and Flow in Trade Unionism. New York: National Bureau of Economic Research, 1936.

B. SECONDARY SOURCES

Abrams, Philip. "The Failure of Social Reform, 1918-1920." Past and Present 24 (1963): 43-64.

Adams, Paul. "Social Control or Social Wage: On the Political Economy of the 'Welfare State.'" Journal of Sociology and Social Welfare 5 (1978): 46-54.

Addison, Paul. The Road to 1945: British Politics and the Second World War. London: Jonathan Cape, 1975.

Alford, Robert R. Health Care Politics: Ideological and Interest Group Barriers to Reform. Chicago and London: University of Chicago Press, 1975.

_____. "The Political Economy of Health Care: Dynamics Without Change." Politics and Society 2 (1972): 127-64.

Althusser, Louis and Balibar, Etienne. Reading Capital, 2nd ed. London: Schocken Books, 1978.

Altmeyer, Arthur J. The Formative Years of Social Security. Madison: University of Wisconsin Press, 1966.

Altvater, Elmer. "Notes on Some Problems of State Interventionism." Kapitalistate 2 (1973): 76-83.

Andreski, Stanislav. Military Organization and Society, 2nd ed. Berkeley and Los Angeles: University of California Press, 1968.

Bachman, George W. and Meriam, Lewis. The Issue of Compulsory Health Insurance. A Study Prepared at the Request of Senator H. Alexander Smith, chairman of the Subcommittee on Health of the Senate Commitee on Labor and Public Welfare. Washington, D.C.: Brookings Institution, 1948.

Balbus, Isaac D. "The Concept of Interest in Pluralist and Marxian Analysis." Politics and Society 1 (1971): 151-77.

_____. "The Negation of the Negation: Theory of Capitalism Within an Historical Theory of Social Change." Politics and Society 3 (1972): 49-63.

_____. "Politics as Sports." In Leon N. Lindberg et al., eds, Stress and Contradiction in Modern Capitalism: Public Policy and Theory of the State. Lexington, Mass.: Lexington Books, 1975.

_____. "Ruling Elite Theory vs. Marxist Class Analysis." Monthly Review 23 (May 1971): 36-46.

Barker, Colin. "A 'New' Reformism? A Critique of the Political Theory of Nicos Poulantzas." International Socialism, series 2, no. 4 (1979): 88-108.

_____. "The State as Capital." International Socialism, series 2, no. 1 (1978): 16-42.

Bell, Daniel. "The Public Household-On 'Fiscal Sociology' and the Liberal Society." The Public Interest 37 (1974): 29-68.

Benedict, Murray R. Can We Solve the Farm Problem? An Analysis of Federal Aid to Agriculture. New York: The Twentieth Century Fund, 1955.

_____. Farm Policies of the United States 1790-1950: A Study of Their Origins and Development. New York: The Twentieth Century Fund, 1953.

Bernstein, Barton J., ed. Towards a New Past: Dissenting Essays in American History. New York: Random House, 1968.

Bettley, F. Ray. "The Medical Conduct of a Brothel." British Journal of Venereal Diseases 25 (1949): 56-66.

Beveridge, William H. (Lord). Power and Influence. New York: Beechhurst Press, 1955.

Black, John Donald and Kiefer, Maxine Enlow. Future Food and Agricultural Policy. New York: McGraw-Hill Book Co., 1948.

Branson, Noreen and Heinemann, Margot. Britain in the Nineteen Thirties. London: Weidenfeld & Nicolson, 1971.

Bourne, Randolph S. War and the Intellectuals: Collected Essays 1915-1919. Edited with an Introduction by Carl Resek. New York: Harper Torchbooks, Harper & Row, 1964.

Boyer, Richard O. and Morais, Herbert M. Labor's Untold Story. New York: Cameron Associates, 1955.

Briggs, Asa. "The Welfare State in Historical Perspective." Archives Européenes de Sociologie 2 (1961): 221-58.

Bruce, Maurice. The Coming of the Welfare State, 4th ed. London: Batsford, 1968.

Bullock, Alan. The Life and Times of Ernest Bevin. Vol. 1: Trade Union Leader. London: Heinemann, 1960, Vol. 2: Minister of Labour. London: Heinemann, 1967.

Burnett, John. Plenty and Want: A Social History of Diet in England from 1815 to the Present Day. London: Nelson, 1966.

Burridge, T.D. British Labour and Hitler's War. London: André Deutsch, 1976.

Calder, Angus. The People's War: Britain 1939-45, 2nd ed. London: Panther Books, 1971.

Callinicos, Alex. Althusser's Marxism. London: Pluto Press, 1976.

Campbell, Douglas J. "Venereal Diseases in the Armed Forces Overseas (2)." British Journal of Venereal Diseases 22 (1946): 158-64.

Capeci, Dominic J., Jr. The Harlem Riot of 1943. Philadelphia: Temple University Press, 1977.

Chadwick, Henry D., M.D. and Pope, Alton S., M.D. The Modern Attack on Tuberculosis. Rev. ed. New York: The Commonwealth Fund, 1946.

Chafe, William F. The American Woman: Her Changing Social, Economic, and Political Roles, 1920-1970. New York: Oxford University Press, 1972.

Chamberlin, Eric R. Life in Wartime Britain. London: Batsford, 1972.

Chester, Daniel N., ed. Lessons of the British War Economy. National Institute of Economic and Social Research. Economic and Social Studies, vol. 10. Cambridge: Cambridge University Press, 1951.

Clark, F. Le Gros. Social History of the School Meals Service. National Council of Social Service: London, 1948.

Clarkson, Kenneth W. Food Stamps and Nutrition. With a Foreword by Yale Brozen. Washington, D.C.: American Enterprise Institute for Public Policy Research, 1975.

Cliff, Tony. The Crisis: Social Contract or Socialism. London: Pluto Press for Socialist Worker, 1975.

Clynes, John R. Memoirs. London: Hutchinson, 1937.

Cochrane, A. L. Effectiveness and Efficiency: Random Reflections on Health Services. Abingdon, England: Nuffield Provincial Hospitals Trust: 1972.

Cole, G.D.H. History of the Labour Party since 1914. London: Routledge & Kegan Paul, 1948.

Coller, F.H. A State Trading Adventure. London: Oxford University Press, H. Milford, 1925.

Coppock, Joseph D. "The Food Stamp Plan." Transactions of the American Philosophical Society, 37, pt. 2 (1947): 131-200. Published by Lancaster Press (Lancaster, Pa.).

Cowling, Maurice. The Impact of Hitler: British Politics and British Policy 1933-1940. London: Cambridge University Press, 1975.

Corea, Gena. The Hidden Malpractice: How American Medicine Treats Women as Patients and Professionals. New York: Morrow, 1977.

Crew, Francis Albert Eley, F.R.S., ed. The Army Medical Services. Administration, Vol. 2. History of the Second World War, United Kingdom Medical Series. London: H.M.S.O., 1955.

Crouch, Colin. "Varieties of Trade Union Weakness: Organized Labour and Capital Formation in Britain, Federal Germany and Sweden." West European Politics 3 (1980): 87-106.

Cummings, Richard Osborn. The American and HIs Food: A History of Food Habits in the United States. Rev. ed. Chicago: University of Chicago Press, 1941.

Cutler, John C. "Role of Prophylaxis and Education in Venereal Disease Control." In International Venereal Disease Symposium. 2nd, St. Louis, 1972. Epidemic: Venereal Disease. Miami: Symposia Specialists, 1973.

Dahrendorf, Ralf. Class and Class Conflict in Industrial Societies. Translated, revised, and expanded by the author. Stanford, Calif.: Stanford University Press, 1959.

Dalrymple-Champneys, Sir Weldon. "The Epidemiological Control of Venereal Disease." British Journal of Venereal Diseases 23 (1947): 101-5.

Davis, Howard P. "Sharing Our Bounty." In Food: The Yearbook of Agriculture 1959. Washington, D.C.: United States Department of Agriculture, 1959, pp. 681-90.

Dean, Basil. The Theatre at War. London: Harrap, 1956.

De Caux, Len. Labor Radical: A Personal History. Boston: Beacon, 1970.

Dobbs, Farrell. Teamster Rebellion. New York: Monad Press for the Anchor Foundation, Inc., 1972.

Draper, Hal. Karl Marx's Theory of Revolution. Vol. 1. State and Bureaucracy. New York and London: Monthly Review Press, 1977.

_____. "Neo-Corporatists and Neo-Reformers." New Politics 1, no. 1 (1961): 87-106.

Dratch, Howard. "The Politics of Child Care in the 1940s." Science and Society 38 (1974): 167-204.

Drummond, Jack C. and Wilbraham, Anne. The Englishman's Food: A History of Five Centuries of English Diet. Rev. ed. London: Jonathan Cape, 1957.

Dubos, Rene. Mirage of Health: Utopias, Progress, and Biological Change. Perennial Library edition. New York: Harper & Row, 1971.

Dubos, René and Jean. The White Plague: Tuberculosis, Man and Society. Boston: Little, Brown & Co., 1952.

Easton, David. The Political System: An Inquiry into the State of Political Science. New York: Knopf, 1953.

Eckstein, Harry. The English Health Service: Its Origins, Structure, and Achievements. Cambridge, Mass.: Harvard University Press, 1958.

Edelman, Murray. Symbolic Uses of Politics. Urbana: University of Illinois Press, 1964.

Fenelon, K.G. Britain's Food Supplies. London: Methuen, 1952.

Ferguson, Sheila and Fitzgerald, Hilde. Studies in the Social Services. History of the Second World War, United Kingdom Civil Series. London: H.M.S.O. and Longmans, Green & Co., 1954.

Fine, Ben and Harris, Laurence. "'State Expenditure in Advanced Capitalism': A Critique." New Left Review 98 (1976): 96-112.

Fitz Gibbon, Constantine. The Blitz. With drawings by Henry Moore. London: Allan Wingate, 1957.

Flanagan, Thelma G. "School Food Services." In Fuller, Edgar and Pearson, Jim B., eds, Education in the States: Nationwide Development Since 1900. A Project of the Chief State School Officers. Washington, D. C.: National Education Association, 1969, pp. 555-610.

Foner, Philip S. Organized Labor and the Black Worker. New York: Praeger, 1974.

Foot, Michael. Aneurin Bevan. Vol. 1: 1897-1945. London: Mac-Gibbon & Kee, 1962. Vol. 2: 1945-1960. London, Davis-Poynter, 1973.

Foot, Paul, The Politics of Harold Wilson. Harmondsworth, England: Penguin Books, 1968.

Foster, William. John Company. London: John Lane, 1926.

Foucault, Michel. The History of Sexuality. Vol. 1. Translated by Robert Hurtley. New York: Pantheon, 1978.

Fox, Daniel. "Social Policy and City Politics:" Tuberculosis Reporting in New York, 1889-1900." Bulletin of the History of Medicine 49 (1975): 169-95.

Francis, John. Bovine Tuberculosis. London: Staples Press, 1947.

Fraser, Derek. The Evolution of the British Welfare State: A History of Social Policy since the Industrial Revolution. London and Basingstoke: Macmillan, 1973.

Frazer, William M. A History of English Public Health 1834-1939. London: Bailliere, Tindall & Cox, 1950.

Freeman, Roger. The Growth of American Government: A Morphology of the Welfare State. Stanford, Calif.: Hoover Institution Press, Stanford University, 1975.

Furniss, Norman. "The Welfare Debate in Great Britain: Implications for the United States." Public Administration Review 35 (1975): 300-09.

Furniss, Norman and Tilton, Timothy. The Case for the Welfare State: From Social Security to Social Equality. Bloomington and London: Indiana University Press, 1977.

Garraty, John A. "The New Deal, National Socialism, and the Great Depression." American Historical Review 78 (1973): 907-44.

Giddens, Anthony. The Class Structure of the Advanced Societies. London: Hutchinson, 1973.

Gilbert, Bentley B. British Social Policy 1918-1939. London: Batsford, 1970.

Glazer, Nathan. "The Limits of Social Policy." Commentary 52, No. 3(1971): 51-58.

Gough, Ian. The Political Economy of the Welfare State. London and Basingstoke: Macmillan, 1979.

_____. "State Expenditures in Advanced Capitalism." New Left Review 92 (1975): 53-92.

_____. "Theories of the Welfare State: A Critique." International Journal of Health Services 8 (1978): 27-40.

Graham, Otis L., Jr. Toward A Planned Society: From Roosevelt to Nixon. New York: Oxford University Press, 1976.

Green, James. "Fighting on Two Fronts: Working-Class Militancy in the 1940's." Radical America 9, nos. 4-5 (1975): 7-47.

Greenberg, Edward S. Serving the Few: Corporate Capitalism and the Bias of Government Policy. New York: Wiley, 1974.

Gusfield, Joseph R. Symbolic Crusade: Status Politics and the American Temperance Movement. Urbana, Illinois: University of Illinois Press, 1973.

Habermas, Jurgen. Legitimation Crisis. Translated by Thomas McCarthy. Boston: Beacon Press, 1975.

Hall, Ben. "Labor Policy: New Deal and Fair Deal, Tracing the Trend Toward State Controls." New International 15 (1949): 163-67.

Hamby, Alonzo L. "Sixty Million Jobs and the People's Revolution: The Liberals, the New Deal and World War II." Historian 30 (1968): 578-98.

Hammond, R.J. Food. Vol. 1: The Growth of Policy; Vols. 2-3: Studies in Administration and Control. History of the Second World War, United Kingdom Civil Series. London: H.M.S.O. and Longmans, Green & Co., 1951, 1962.

_____. Food and Agriculture in Britain 1939-45: Aspects of Wartime Control. Food Research Institute, Stanford, Calif.: Stanford University Press, 1954.

Hancock, William Keith and Gowing, Margaret M. The British War Economy. History of the Second World War. United Kingdom Civil Series. London: H.M.S.O., 1949.

Hardin, Charles M. The Politics of Agriculture: Soil Conservation and the Struggle for Power in Rural America. Glencoe, Ill.: Free Press, 1952

Harris, Jose. "Social Planning in War-Time: Some Aspects of the Beveridge Report." In Winter, J.M., ed., War and Economic Development, Cambridge: Cambridge University Press, 1975.

_____. William Beveridge: A Biography. Oxford: Clarendon Press, 1977.

Harris, Nigel. Competition and the Corporate Society: British Conservatives, the State and Industry 1945-1964. London: Methuen, 1972.

_____. "The Decline of Welfare." International Socialism, series 1, 7 (1961): 5-14.

Harrisson, Tom. Living Through the Blitz. London: Collins, 1976.

Hartwell, R.M. "The Rising Standard of Living in England 1800-50." Economic History Review 13 (1961): 397-416.

Hartzell, Karl Drew. The Empire State at War: World War II. State of New York, 1949.

Havighurst, Robert J. and Morgan, H. Gerthon. The Social History of a War-Boom Community. New York: Longmans, Green, 1951.

Heclo, Hugh. Modern Social Politics in Britain and Sweden: From Relief to Income Maintenance. New Haven and London: Yale University Press, 1974.

Heidenheimer, Arnold. "Politics of Public Education, Health and Welfare in U.S.A. and Western Europe." British Journal of Political Science 3 (1973): 315-40.

Hirsch, Joachim. "The State Apparatus and Social Reproduction: Elements of a Theory of the Bourgeois State." In John Holloway and Sol Piccioto, eds. London: Arnold, 1978.

Hobsbaw, E.J. "The British Standard of Living 1790-1850." In Labouring Man: Studies in the History of Labour. London: Weidenfeld and Nicolson, 1964.

Hofstadter, Richard. The Age of Reform; from Bryan to F.D.R. New York: Knopf, 1955.

Holloway, John and Picciotto, Sol. "Capital, Crisis and the State." Capital and Class 2 (1977): 76-101.

Holloway, John and Picciotto, Sol, eds. State and Capital: A Marxist Debate. London: Edward Arnold, 1978.

Honigsbaum, Frank. The Struggle for the Ministry of Health, 1914-1919. London: Bell, 1970.
Hoos, Ida R. Systems Analysis in Public Policy: A Critique. Berkeley: University of California Press, 1972.

International Labour Office. Nutrition in Industry. Studies and Reports, New Series No. 4. Montreal: International Labour Office, 1946.

_____. War and Women's Employment. Montreal: International Labour Office, 1946.

International Venereal Disease Symposium, 2nd, St. Louis, 1972. Epidemic: Venereal Disease. Sponsored and distributed by Pfizer Laboratories Division, Pfizer Inc., and American Social Health Association. Miami: Symposia Specialists, 1973.

Janeway, Eliot. The Struggle for Survival. New Haven: Yale University Press, 1951.

Jennings, Edward. "Wildcat! The Wartime Strike Wave in Auto." With an Epilogue by Martin Glaberman. Radical America 9, nos. 4-5 (1975): 77-113.

Karabel, Jerome. "The Failure of American Socialism Reconsidered." In Miliband, Ralph and Saville, John, eds, The Socialist Register, London: Merlin Press, 1980.

_____. "The Reasons Why." New York Review of Books 26 (February 1979): 22-27.

Katznelson, Ira. "Considerations on Social Democracy in the United States." Comparative Politics 11 (1978): 77-99.

Kaufman, Arnold S. The Radical Liberal: New Man in American Politics. New York: Atherton Press, 1968.

Kelman, Sander. "Adventure in the Undialectical." In "Stalking the Poiltics of Health Care Reform: Three Critical Perspectives on Robert R. Alford's Health Care Politics: Ideological and Interest Group Barriers to Reform." Journal of Health Politics, Policy and Law I (1976): 122-129.

Kidron, Michael. Capitalism and Theory. London: Pluto Press, 1974.

_____. Western Capitalism Since the War. Rev. ed. Harmondsworth, England: Penguin Books, 1970.

Kincaid, Jim. "The Decline of the Welfare State." In World Crisis: Essays in Revolutionary Socialism, Harris, Nigel and Palmer, John eds., London: Hutchinson, 1972, Chapter 2.

King, Cecil H. With Malice Toward None: A War Diary. London: Sidgwick & Jackson, 1970.

Kirkendall, Richard S., ed. The New Deal: The Historical Debate. New York: Wiley, 1973.

Kristol, Irving. "Taxes, Poverty, and Equality." The Public Interest 37 (1974): 3-28.

Lasagna, Louis. The VD Epidemic: How It Started, Where It's Going, and What to Do About It. Philadelphia: Temple University Press, 1975.

Lees, Robert. "Venereal Diseases in the Armed Forces Overseas (1)." British Journal of Venereal Diseases 22 (1946): 149-58.

Leiby, James. A History of Social Welfare and Social Work in the United States. New York: Columbia University Press, 1978.

Lehmann, John. I Am My Brother: Autobiography II. London: Longmans, 1959.

Lens, Sidney, The Labor Wars: From the Molly Maguires to the Sitdowns. Garden City, N.Y.: Doubleday, 1973.

Lerner, Monroe and Anderson, Odin W. Health Progress in the United States 1900-60. A Report of Health Information Foundation. Chicago & London: University of Chicago Press, 1963.

Leuchtenberg, William E. "The New Deal and the Analogue of War." In Braeman, John, Bremner, Robert H., and Walters, Everett eds., Change and Continuity in Twentieth Century America. Columbus: Ohio State University Press, 1964, pp. 81-143.

Lichtenstein, Nelson. "Defending the No-Strike Pledge: CIO Politics During World War II." Radical America 9, nos. 4-5 (1975): 49-75.

Lindberg, Leon N., Alford, Robert, Crouch, Colin and Offe, Claus, eds. Stress and Contradiction in Modern Capitalism: Public Policy and the Theory of the State. Lexington, Mass.: Lexington Books, 1975.

Lingeman, Richard R. Don't You Know There's a War On? The American Home Front, 1941-1945. New York: G.P. Putnam's Sons, 1970.

Lloyd, Trevor O. Empire to Welfare State: English History 1906-1967. London: Oxford University Press. 1970.

Longmate, Norman. The GIs: The Americans in Britain 1942-1945. New York: Scribner, 1975.

Lowell, Anthony. Tuberculosis. Cambridge, Mass.: Harvard University Press, 1969.

Ludendorff, Erich von. My War Memories, 1914-1918. 2nd ed. London: Hutchinson, 1920.

McConnell, Grant. Private Power and American Democracy. New York: Knopf, 1966.

McDougall, J.B. Tuberculosis: A Global Study in Social Pathology. Edinburgh: E. & S. Livingstone, 1950.

McKeown, Thomas. Medicine in Modern Society: Medical Planning Based on Evaluation of Medical Achievement. New York: Hafner, 1966.

_____. The Role of Medicine: Dream, Mirage, or Nemesis? Princeton, N.J.: Princeton University Press, 1979.

MacNalty, Sir Arthur Salusbury, ed. The Civilian Health and Medical Services. vol. 1. The Ministry of Health Services: Other Civilian Health and Medical Services. History of the Second World War, United Kingdom Medical Series. London: H.M.S.O., 1953.

MacNalty, Sir Arthur Salusbury and Mellor, W. Franklin. Medical Services in War: The Principal Medical Lessons of the Second World War. History of the Second World War, United Kingdom Medical Series. London: H.M.S.O., 1968.

Marrack, J.R. "Investigations of Human Nutrition in the United Kingdom during the War." Proceedings of the Nutrition Society 5 (1947): 213-41.

Martin, Kingsley. Harold Laski, 1893-1950: A Biographical Memoir. London: Gollancz, 1953.

Marwick, Arthur. Britain in the Century of Total War: War Peace and Social Change 1900-1967. London: The Bodley Head, 1968.

_____. "The Labour Party and the Welfare State in Britain, 1900-1948." American Historical Review 73 (1967): 380-403.

_____. War and Social Change in the Twentieth Century: A Comparative Study of Britain, France, Germany, Russia and the United States. London and Basingstoke: Macmillan, 1974.

Merrill, Francis E. Social Problems on the Home Front: A Study of War-Time Influences. New York: Harper & Brothers, 1948.

Miliband, Ralph. "Lenin's The State and Revolution." In Miliband, Ralph and Saville, John, eds., Socialist Register 1970, Merlin Press, 1970, pp. 309-19.

_____. "Marx and the State." In Miliband, Ralph and Savile, John, eds., Socialist Register 1965. London: Merlin Press, 1965, pp. 278-96.

_____. Parliamentary Socialism: A Study in the Politics of Labour. London: Merlin Press, 1973.

_____. "Poulantzas and the Capitalist State." New Left Review 82 (1973): 83-92.

_____. "Reply to Nicos Poulantzas." New Left Review 59 (1970): 53-60.

_____. The State in Capitalist Society. London: Weidenfeld & Nicolson, 1969.

Mills, C. Wright. Power, Politics and People: The Collected Essays of C. Wright Mills. Edited and with an introduction by Irving Louis Horowitz. New York: Oxford University Press, 1963.

Milward, Alan S. The Economic Effects of the Two World Wars on Britain. Prepared for the Economic History Society. London and Basingstoke: Macmillan, 1970.

_____. War, Economy and Society, 1939-1945. London: Allen Lane, Penguin Books, 1977.

Mitchell, Juliet. Psychoanalysis and Feminism. New York: Pantheon, 1974.

Mowat, Charles Loch. Britain Between the Wars 1918-1940. Chicago: University of Chicago Press, 1955.

Murray, Keith A.H. Agriculture. History of the Second World War, United Kingdom Civil Series. London: H.M.S.O. and Longmans, Green & Co., 1955.

Myrdal, Gunnar. Beyond the Welfare State: Economic Planning and Its International Implications. New Haven and London: Yale University Press, 1960.

Nash, E.F. "Wartime Control of Food and Agricultural Prices." In Chester, D.N., ed., Lessons of the British War Economy. National Institute of Economic and Social Research. Cambridge: Cambridge University Press, 1951.

Navarro, Vicente. Class Struggle, the State and Medicine: An Historical and Contemporary Analysis of the Medical Sector in Great Britain. New York: Prodist, 1978.

Nelson, Keith L., ed. The Impact of War on American Life: The Twentieth-Century Experience. New York: Holt, Rinehart & Winston, 1971.

Newberne, P.M. and Williams, G. "Nutritional Influences on the Course of Infections." In Dunlop, R.H. and Moon, H.W., eds., Resistance to Infectious Disease. Saskatoon: Saskatoon Modern Press, 1970.

Nielander, William A. Wartime Food Rationing in the United States. Ottawa and Washington, D.C.: World Trade Relations, 1947.

Nixon, Edgar B., ed. Franklin D. Roosevelt and Conservation, 1911-1945. 2 vols. Washington, D.C.: Government Printing Office, 1957.

O'Connor, James. The Fiscal Crisis of the State. New York: St. Martin's Press, 1973.

Offe, Claus. "The Abolition of Market Control and the Problem of Legitimacy." Part 1. Kapitalistate 1 (1973): 109-16. Part 2. Kapitalistate 2 (1973): 73-75.

_____. "Advanced Capitalism and the Welfare State." Politics and Society 2 (1972): 479-88.

Ollman, Bertell. Social and Sexual Revolution: Essays on Marx and Reich. Boston: South End Press, 1979.

Olson, Mancur, Jr. The Economics of the Wartime Shortage: A History of British Food Supplies in the Napoleonic War and in World Wars I and II. Durham, N.C.: Duke University Press, 1963.

Oppenheimer, Valerie Kincade. The Female Labor Force in the United States: Demographic and Economic Factors Governing Its Growth and Changing Composition. Berkeley: University of California Press, 1972. Organization for Economic Cooperation and Development. Expenditure Trends in OECD Countries. Paris: OECD, 1972.

Orr, John Boyd. As I Recall. With an introduction by Ritchie Calder. Garden City, N.Y.: Doubleday, 1967.

Osmond, T.E. "Venereal Disease in Peace and War, with Some Reminiscences of the Last Forty Years." British Journal of Venereal Diseases 25 (1949): 101-114.

Paarlberg, Don. Subsidized Food Consumption. Washington, D.C., American Enterprise Institute, 1963.

Panitch, Leo. Social Democracy and Industrial Militancy: The Labour Party, the Trade Unions and Incomes Policy, 1945-1974. Cambridge: Cambridge University Press, 1976.

Parker, Henry, M.D. Manpower: A Study of War-Time Policy and Administration. History of the Second World War, United Kingdom Civil Series. London: H.M.S.O. and Longmans, Green & Co., 1957.

Peacock, Alan T. and Wiseman, Jack, assisted by Jindrich Veverka. The Growth of Public Expenditure in the United Kingdom. Rev. ed. London: Allen & Unwin, 1967.

Pelling, Henry. Britain and the Second World War. London: Collins, 1970.

_____. The British Communist Party. London: Adam & Charles Black, 1958.

_____. History of British Trade Unionism. London: Macmillan, 1963.

_____. Popular Politics and Society in Late Victorian England. London: Fontana, 1968.

_____. A Short History of the Labour Party. London: Macmillan, 1968.

Perlman, Selig. A Theory of the Labor Movement. New York: Augustus M. Kelley, 1928.

Perrett, Geoffrey. Days of Sadness, Years of Triumph: The American People 1939-1945. New York: Coward, McCann & Geoghegan, Inc., 1973.

Piven, Frances Fox and Cloward, Richard A. Regulating the Poor: The Function of Public Welfare. New York: Random House, 1971.

Polenberg, Richard. War and Society: The United States, 1941-1945. Philadelphia, New York, Toronto: J.B. Lippincott Company, 1972.

Porter, Bruce D. "Parkinson's Law Revisited: War and the Growth of Government." The Public Interest 60 (1980): 50-68.

Postan, Michael M. British War Production. History of the Second World War, United Kingdom Civil Series. London: H.M.S.O., 1952.

Potter, Jim. The American Economy Between the World Wars. London and Basingstoke: Macmillan, 1974.

Poulantzas, Nicos. Classes in Contemporary Capitalism. Translated by David Fernbach. London: Verso, 1978.

_____. "On Social Classes." New Left Review 78 (1974): 27-55.

_____. Political Power and Social Classes. Translated by Timothy O'Hagan. London: NLB and Sheed & Ward, 1973.

_____. "The Problem of the Capitalist State." New Left Review 58 (1969): 67-78. Reprinted in Blackburn, Robin, ed., Ideology in Social Science. London: Fontana, 1972, pp. 238-62.

_____. State, Power, Socialism. Translated by Patrick Camiller. London: NLB, 1978.

Powles, John. "On the Limitations of Modern Medicine." Science, Medicine, and Man 1, no. 1 (1973): 1-30.

Preis, Art. Labor's Giant Step: Twenty Years of the CIO. New York: Pioneer Publishers. 1964.

Radical America 9, nos. 4-5 (1974). Special issue on "American Labor in the 1940's."

Rankin, William. "What Dunkirk Spirit?" New Society 26 (1973): 396-98.

Rayback, Joseph. A History of American Labor. New York: Free Press, 1966.

Rexford-Welch, Squadron Leader S.C., ed. The Royal Air Force Medical Services. Vol. 2: Administration. History of the Second World War, United Kingdom Medical Series. London: H.M.S.O., 1954.

Rimlinger, Gaston V. "Welfare Policy and Economic Development: A Comparative Historical Perspective." Journal of Economic History 26 (1966): 556-71.

_____. Welfare Policy and Industrialization in Europe, America, and Russia. New York: John Wiley & Sons, 1971.

Robinson, Paul A. The Freudian Left: Wilhelm Reich, Geza Roheim, Herbert Marcuse. New York: Harper & Row, 1969.

Roll, Eric. The Combined Food Board: A Study in Wartime International Planning. Food Research Institute. Stanford, Calif.: Stanford University Press, 1956.

Rolph, C.H., ed. Women of the Streets: A Sociological Study of the Common Prostitute. Edited for and on behalf of the British Social Biology Council. London: Secker & Warburg, 1955.

Romanyshyn, John M., with the assistance of Annie L. Romanyshyn. Social Welfare: Charity to Justice. New York: Random House, 1971.

Rosen, George. A History of Public Health. New York: M.D. Publications, 1958.

Rosen, S. McKee. The Combined Boards of the Second World War: An Experiment in International Administration. New York: Columbia University Press, 1951.

Ross, Davis R.B. Preparing for Ulysses: Politics and Veterans During World War II. New York and London: Columbia University Press, 1969.

Salter, James Arthur (Lord). Allied Shipping Control: An Experiment in International Administration. Oxford: Clarendon Press; London, New York: Milford, 1921.

Sandstrom, Marvin M. "School Lunches." In Food: The Yearbook of Agriculture 1959. Washington, D.C.: United States Department of Agriculture, 1959: 691-700.

Schottland, Charles I., ed. The Welfare State. New York: Harper & Row, 1967.

Seidman, Joel. American Labor from Defense to Reconversion. Chicago: University of Chicago Press, 1953.

Shannon, Fred Albert. America's Economic Growth, 3d ed. New York: Macmillan, 1951.

Shonfield, Andrew. Modern Capitalism: The Changing Balance of Public and Private Power. London: Oxford University Press for the Royal Institute of International Affairs, 1965.

Shryock, Richard Harrison. National Tuberculosis Association 1904-1954: A Study of the Voluntary Health Movement in the United States. New York: National Tuberculosis Association, 1957.

Sigerist, Henry E. "War and Medicine." In Roemer, Milton I., ed., Henry E. Sigerist on the Sociology of Medicine. New York: M.D. Publications, 1960, pp. 337-47.

Sitkoff, Harvard. "Racial Militancy and Interracial Violence in the Second World War." Journal of American History 58 (1971): 661-81.

Solomon, Saul, M.D. Tuberculosis. New York: Coward-McCann, 1952.

Sombart, Werner. Why Is There No Socialism in the United States? Translated by Patricia M. Hocking and C.T. Husbands. White Plains, N.Y.: M.E. Sharpe, 1976.

Somers, Gerald G., ed. Labor, Management, and Social Policy: Essays in the John R. Commons Tradition. Madison: University of Wisconsin Press, 1963.

Somers, Herman Miles and Somers, Anne Ramsay. Doctors, Patients and Health Insurance: The Organization and Financing of Medical Care. Washington, D.C.: Brookings Institution, 1961.

Steiner, Gilbert Y. The State of Welfare. Washington, D.C.: The Brookings Institution, 1971.

Stevenson, John. Social Conditions in Britain Between the Wars. Harmondsworth, England: Penguin Books, 1977.

Stinchcombe, Arthur L. Theoretical Methods in Social History. New York, San Francisco, London: Academic Press, 1978.

Thomas, Hugh. John Strachey. London: Harper & Row, 1973.

Thompson, E.P. "A Question of Manners." New Society 27 (1974): 91-2.

Thompson, Laurence. 1940. New York: William Morrow & Co., 1966.

Titmuss, Richard M. Commitment to Welfare. London: George Allen & Unwin, 1968.

_____. Essays on "The Welfare State," 2nd ed. London: Unwin University Books, George Allen & Unwin, 1963.

_____. Problems of Social Policy. History of the Second World War, United Kingdom Civil Series. London: H.M.S.O. and Longmans, Green & Co., 1950.

186 / HEALTH OF THE STATE

_____. Social Policy: An Introduction. Edited by Brian Abel-Smith and Kay Titmuss. London: George Allen & Unwin, 1974.

Todhunter, Elizabeth Neige. "The Story of Nutrition." In Food: The Yearbook of Agriculture 1959. Washington, D.C.: United States Department of Agriculture, 1959: 7-22.

Trattner, Walter I. From Poor Law to Welfare State: A History of Social Welfare in America, 2nd ed. New York: The Free Press, 1979.

Trey, Joan Ellen. "Women in the War Economy — World War II." Review of Radical Political Economics 4, 3 (1973): 40-57.

Trotsky, Leon. The History of the Russian Revolution. Translated by Max Eastman. New York: Simon & Schuster, 1932.

_____. 1905. Translated by Anya Bostock. New York: Random House, 1971.

_____. On the Labor Party in the United States. New York: Pathfinder Press, 1967.

United Kingdom. Central Statistical Office. Annual Abstract of Statistics, no. 86, 1938-1948. London: H.M.S.O., 1949.

_____. Statistical Digest of the War. London: H.M.S.O., 1951.

United Kingdom. Ministry of Food. How Britain Was Fed in Wartime. Food Control, 1939-1945. London: H.M.S.O., 1946.

United Kingdom. Ministry of Health. On the State of the Public Health During Six Years of War. Report of the Chief Medical Officer of the Ministry of Health, 1939-45. London: H.M.S.O., 1946.

United States Army. Medical Department. Preventive Medicine in World War II. Vol. 5: Communicable Diseases Transmitted Through Contact by Unknown Means. Washington, D.C.: Office of the Surgeon General, Department of the Army, 1960.

_____. Preventive Medicine in World War II. Vol. 8: Civil Affairs/ Military Government Public Health Activities. Washington, D.C.: Office of the Surgeon General, Department of the Army, 1976.

United States. Bureau of the Budget. The United States at War: Development and Administration of the War Program by the

Federal Government. Historical Reports on War Administration. Bureau of the Budget No. 1. Washington, D.C.: Government Printing Office, 1946.

United States. Bureau of the Census. Historical Statistics of the United States: Colonial Times to 1970. Bicentenial Edition. Part I. Washington, D.C.: Government Printing Office, 1976.

Veblen, Thorstein. Absentee Ownership and Business Enterprise in Recent Times: The Case of America. New York: B.W. Huebsch, 1923.

Vogel, David. "Why Businessmen Distrust Their State." British Journal of Political Science 8 (1978): 45-78.

Vonderlehr, Raymond A. and Heller, J.R. The Control of Venereal Disease. New York: Reynal & Hitchcock, 1946.

Walkowitz, Judith R. Prostitution and Victorian Society: Women, Class, and the State. Cambridge: Cambridge University Press, 1980.

Ward, Matthew. Indignant Heart. New York: New Books, 1952.

Watt, Muriel G. "The Development of the School Meals Scheme." British Journal of Nutrition 2 (1948): 77-81.

Wedderburn, Dorothy. "Facts and Theories of the Welfare State." In Miliband, Ralph and Saville, John, eds., Socialist Register 1965. London: Merlin Press, 1965, pp. 127-46.

Weinstein, James. The Corporate Ideal in the Liberal State. Boston: Beacon Press, 1968.

Weinstein, James and Eakins, David W., eds., For a New America: Essays in History and Politics from Studies on the Left, 1959-1967. New York: Vintage, 1970.

Wildavsky, Aaron. "Doing Better and Feeling Worse: The Political Pathology of Health Policy." In Knowles, John H., M.D., ed. Doing Better and Feeling Worse: Health in the United States. New York: W.W. Norton, 1977.

Wilensky, Harold. The "New Corporatism," Centralization, and the Welfare State. Beverly Hills, CA: Sage Publications, 1976.

_____. The Welfare State and Equality: Structural and Ideological Roots of Public Expenditures. Berkeley, Los Angeles, London: University of California Press, 1975.

Wilensky, Harold and Lebeaux, Charles N. Industrial Society and Social Welfare. Rev. ed. New York: Free Press, 1965.

Willcox, R.R. "Prostitution and Venereal Disease: Proportion of Venereal Disease Acquired from Prostitutes in Asia: A Comparison with France, the United Kingdom, and the United States of America." British Journal of Venereal Diseases 38 (1962): 37-42.

Willcox, R.R. "Prostitution and Venereal Disease: Social Considerations of Prostitution." British Journal of Preventive Social Medicine 15 (1961): 42-47.

Winant, John G. Letter from Grosvenor Square: An Account of a Stewardship. Boston: Houghton Mifflin Co., 1947.

Winter, J.M. "Infant Mortality, Maternal Mortality, and Public Health in Britain in the 1930s." Journal of European Economic History 5 (1979): 439-62.

Winter, J.M., ed. War and Economic Development: Essays in Memory of David Joslin. Cambridge: Cambridge University Press, 1975.

Wolfe, Alan. The Limits of Legitimacy. New York: Free Press, 1977.

Woolton, Frederick, Earl of. The Memoirs of the Rt. Hon. the Earl of Woolton C.H.,P.C., D. L., LL.D. London: Cassel, 1959.

Wright, Erik Olin. Class, Crisis and State. London: NLB, 1978.

Wynn, Neil A. The Afro-American and the Second World War. London: Paul Elek, 1976.

_____. "The Impact of World War II on the American Negro." Journal of Contemporary History 6 (1971): 42-53.

INDEX

ABOUT THE AUTHOR

PAUL ADAMS is Associate Professor of Social Work at The University of Iowa. From 1975 to 1979 he was Assistant Professor at the School of Social Work, University of Texas at Austin.

Dr. Adams's research is in the area of American and European social policy. His articles and reviews have appeared in <u>Social Service Review</u>, the <u>Journal of Social Policy</u>, the <u>Journal of Sociology and Social Welfare</u>, <u>Contemporary Sociology</u>, and <u>Catalyst</u>.

Dr. Adams holds a B.A. from University College, Oxford, an M.S.W. from the University of Sussex, and a Dip. Soc. Admin. from the London School of Economics. He received his doctorate in social welfare from the University of California, Berkeley.